Helpers in Childbirth

SERIES IN HEALTH CARE FOR WOMEN
Series Editor: **Phyllis Noerager Stern**, DNS, RN, FAAN

Helpers in Childbirth: Midwifery Today Oakley and Houd

In Preparation

Silent Sisters: An Ethnography of Homeless Women Russell

Helpers in Childbirth
Midwifery Today

Ann Oakley
Susanne Houd

Published on behalf of the
World Health Organization,
Regional Office for Europe
by Hemisphere Publishing Corporation

● HEMISPHERE PUBLISHING CORPORATION
A member of the Taylor & Francis Group
New York   Washington   Philadelphia   London

HELPERS IN CHILDBIRTH: Midwifery Today

This book was set in Times Roman by Hemisphere Publishing Corporation. The editors were Lys Ann Shore and Carolyn V. Ormes; the production supervisor was Peggy M. Rote; and the typesetter was Phoebe A. Carter.
Cover design by Debra Eubanks Riffe. Printing and binding by BookCrafters, Inc.

A CIP catalog record for this book is available from the British Library.

Library of Congress Cataloging-in-Publication Data

Oakley, Ann.
  Helpers in childbirth: midwifery today / Ann Oakley and Susanne Houd.
    p.   cm.
  "Published on behalf of the World Health Organization, Regional Office for Europe by Hemisphere Publishing Corporation."
  Includes bibliographical references (p.
    1. Midwives—History—20th century.   2. Midwives—History.   3. Childbirth—History.   I.
Houd, Susanne.   II. Title.
RG950.023   1990
618.2—dc20   89-26897
                                                                                                    CIP

ISBN 1-56032-036-2
ISSN 1047-4005

Midwife . . . substantive, Middle English (probably formed from MID, preposition + WIFE in the sense 'woman' (so midwoman, thirteenth century), the notion being 'a woman who is *with* the mother at birth.'
Oxford English Dictionary

Contents

Foreword

At the annual meeting of the thirty-two Member States of the European Region of the World Health Organization (WHO) in 1979, the Regional Office was asked to evaluate maternity services and make recommendations. In the process of evaluating these services, it became clear that midwifery services are an essential component of care that is being sorely neglected. Midwifery services are essential because the nature of the care provided by midwives is qualitatively quite different from the care given by obstetricians, although both professions contribute equally important components of care. Surveys suggest that when midwifery is subservient to obstetrics, or is altogether absent, the proper balance in maternity care is lost. This may lead to excessive use of technology and dehumanization of care.

Because the evaluation showed the importance of midwifery to quality maternity care, the WHO Regional Office for Europe decided to launch a research project to attempt to delineate further the nature of midwifery. Susanne Houd, a Danish midwife, and Ann Oakley, an English medical sociologist, had done an outstanding job on a WHO research project on alternative perinatal services, and we asked them to carry out this project. A practicing midwife with wide experience in many care settings together with a sociologist who had spent many years researching and publishing on women's issues and birth issues proved to be an excellent combination for this type of research.

This book is the result of the research project on the nature of midwifery care. Research on midwives has been rare in the past. The information presented here can make a contribution to the important effort to strengthen midwifery and its central role in all maternity care.

J.E. Asvall
Regional Director
WHO Regional Office for Europe
Copenhagen, Denmark

Preface

This book began as a research project that changed its size and character during its gestation period. It is the product of collaborative work both within and outside the World Health Organization (WHO), which has spanned some six years. Ann Oakley is an English sociologist researching and writing in the field of health care and family life, and Susanne Houd is a Danish midwife practicing in both the community and the hospital and also involved in research. Both of us have worked as consultants for WHO, and we are both strongly committed to the idea of international and interdisciplinary work as the only reliable way of escaping from misleadingly narrow frameworks and cultural preoccupations. Midwifery is an international issue. Because childbirth both unites and divides cultures, the issues that preoccupy midwives working in one country will not be far from the heads and hands of others working elsewhere.

Over the past thirty years, a revolution has taken place in the care given to pregnant and birthing women in industrialized countries. Twenty years ago, most deliveries occurred at home, and in most places it was very difficult to obtain a delivery bed in a hospital. Care was mostly given by midwives, and there were few medical interventions in pregnancy or during delivery.

Beginning in the late 1960s, the centralization, medicalization, and technologization of pregnancy and delivery have increased enormously. During the 1970s, the rate of home births dropped considerably in most European countries—even in the Netherlands, famous for its tradition of home-delivered babies. By the end of the 1970s, it had become as difficult to get a home birth as it had previously been to arrange a hospital birth. Through health personnel, the media, and—after a while—friends, relatives, and the community as a whole, the message given to the expectant mother took on a newly ominous tone: birth became an abnormal and therefore dangerous event.

By this time, of course, deaths of mothers and babies had become much rarer than they had ever been. However, labels of normality or abnormality have little to do with the real risks of childbirth. Other factors are important in shaping how childbirth is seen and treated at any particular time. Over much of the industrialized world in the past twenty years, the dominant ideology has become that birth is normal only in retrospect: because of this, hospital birth with all its attendant "in case" technology is said to be the safest kind of birth to have. New rules for birth have been laid down: no birth more than eight hours, no second stage longer than one hour, all women to have episiotomies to prevent prolapse of the uterus in later life, and so on. As an integral part of all these developments, maternity care has come to be more and more under the control of obstetricians, and midwives have found themselves less and less able to care for childbearing women as independent practitioners skilled in the art (or science) of normal childbirth.

The experience of birth as normal has almost disappeared from industrialized society. Over the same period of time, the developed world has moved toward emphasizing the risks and hazards of life in other ways. The constant fear of nuclear war and the experiences of unemployment, crime, pollution, and stress are factors in our daily lives that color all our expectations of what life has to offer. We have lost the ability to look at life positively, concentrating instead on its dangers and risks.

However, social change has a tendency to generate its own counteractions. At the end of the 1960s, another set of attitudes began to emerge. These attitudes are based on a less materialistic lifestyle, on political movements for self-help and personal liberation, and on the idea that life is more likely to be a positive experience if regarded in a positive light. During the 1970s, the extension of this new political awareness into the health care movement spawned grass-roots groups that developed a new model of health care as something communities can and must do for themselves. And, finally, the women's movement and the grass-roots health movement got around to thinking about pregnancy and birth.

At first, the women's movement needed to go through a period of distancing itself from traditional female tasks. Only in the 1980s did it begin to accept that the power lying in the female ability to reproduce can be a source of energy, self-respect, and fulfillment for women. Other groups in the 1970s worked for better birth conditions. These consisted mainly of parents who did not like the births they had had or expected to have and who began to ask awkward questions about the appropriateness, safety, and effectiveness of current birth procedures. Along with feminists and the protagonists of the new models of health care, these groups then began to work in parallel, attempting to retrieve our buried cultural knowledge of normal childbirth.

Increasingly, a confrontation has developed between two models and philosophies of childbearing. In one, pregnancy and birth are areas of life that belong to the medical profession: they are abnormal, disease-like conditions of the body, requiring expert management and control. According to the other model, pregnancy and birth are part of ordinary life experience, even—or especially—because they sometimes merge with death.

Who stands at the point of divergence between these two approaches to childbirth? The midwife. Her legs straddle the chasm between the two philosophies that describe childbirth as medical and social events. She is the expert, but also the practitioner of the normal; her expertise must be channeled into the preservation of the mother as the chief deliverer of her own child. These days, this has become a contradiction in terms, for there is no such thing as normal childbirth any more. The only "normal" childbirths are those that assertive and informed middle-class women fight for—and what can possibly be normal about that?

For these reasons, we have chosen to make midwives the central subject of this book.

In 1981–82, we worked together on a WHO project on alternative perinatal services in Europe and North America, and we prepared a report on this project in 1983. This study was concerned with the alternatives to the official services for pregnancy and birth that existed in ten sample countries (we discuss some of our findings in Chapter 5). Out of this work, ideas developed for further work: interviewing midwives and obstetricians about their definitions of risk in childbirth, and making observations and conducting interviews on the theme of midwifery work, both inside and outside the official services. We were interested in finding out whether midwives and obstetricians tended to differ in their perspectives on childbirth and the mother's role. We wanted to find out what midwives actually did and how their capacity to behave as independent practitioners might be affected by different work settings and ideologies. We do not claim that our research is systematic or representative; it can only offer clues and interpretive insights into the patterns of behavior and attitudes that are the subject of study. Systematic testing of the ideas we present in discussing these data (in Chapter 7) will require much larger samples.

The material collected in this extension of the alternative perinatal services project appears in this book, along with a wide range of other material. The book is a blend of research, secondary material, and "mere" ideas. Its aim is to highlight the role and position of midwives as a key issue in maternity care today.

Fictitious names have been used to protect the privacy of the midwives and pregnant women who were interviewed; portions of these interviews appear throughout the book. We believe that these first-hand accounts emphasize the relevance and immediacy of many of the issues raised in this book.

Aside from our professional qualifications for researching and writing a book of this kind, our own experiences as women and as mothers have given us a driving sense of the importance of birth and of the person who, most of all, is *with* women when they give birth: the midwife.

We thank our friends, our colleagues, our midwives, and our children for contributing in visible and invisible ways to the making of this book. We are particularly grateful to those health professionals providing care for mothers and babies who agreed to be interviewed for the research included in the book, and to all those using and providing such services who allowed us to photograph them or to use photographs taken for their own private use. We acknowledge the services of Johanne Maria Jensen, who graciously offered material from two of her slide shows on birth. Particular debts are owed to Jo Garcia and Marianne Scruggs, who patiently read and advised on the manuscript: but, of course, the final form of the book remains our responsibility.

Ann Oakley
Susanne Houd

Chapter One

What Is a Midwife?

In 1961, the International Confederation of Midwives, the International Federation of Gynecologists and Obstetricians, and the World Health Organization (WHO) jointly defined a midwife. They wrote:

> A midwife is a person who, having been regularly admitted to a midwifery educational programme, duly recognized in the country in which it is located, has successfully completed the prescribed course of studies in midwifery and has acquired the requisite qualifications to be registered and/or legally licensed to practise midwifery. She must be able to give the necessary supervision, care and advice to women during pregnancy, labour and the postpartum period, to conduct deliveries on her own responsibility and to care for the newborn and the infant. This care includes preventive measures, the detection of abnormal conditions in mother and child, the procurement of medical assistance and the execution of emergency measures in the absence of medical help. She has an important task in health counselling and education, not only for the patients but also within the family and the community. The work should involve antenatal education and preparation for parenthood and extends to certain areas of gynaecology, family planning and child

care. She may practise in hospitals, clinics, health units, domiciliary conditions or
in any other service.

Behind this joint definition lie slightly different definitions of midwifery in
different countries. The Swedish definition, for example, states:

> A midwife is a person who is qualified to practice midwifery. She is trained to give
> the necessary care and advice to women during pregnancy, labor, and the postnatal
> period, to conduct normal deliveries on her own responsibility, and to care for the
> newly born infant. At all times, she must be able to recognize the warning signs of
> abnormal conditions that necessitate referral to a doctor, and to carry out emer-
> gency measures in the absence of medical help. She may practice in hospitals,
> health units, or domiciliary services. In any one of these situations, she has an
> important task in health education within the family and the community, family
> planning and child care.

The definition in the Federal Republic of Germany specifies that "the practice
of midwifery includes advice and assistance to pregnant women, supervision
and assistance during delivery and miscarriage, as well as care of lying-in
women and newly born infants." It is stressed that the midwife must deal only
with normal situations. In Italy, the midwife is also responsible for "the surveillance of a mother and her child until the latter has attained the age of three
years."
      Although the wording and the specified period of care differ, the message
is clear: the midwife gives independent care to women who have normal pregnancies and births. Beyond these official definitions of the midwife's role, there
are other important ways of describing her significance to birthing women. For
example, Professor G. J. Kloosterman, former director of the Midwifery
School in Amsterdam, says, "Throughout the world, there exists a group of
women who feel mightily drawn to giving care to women in childbirth. At the
same time maternal and independent, responsive to a mother's needs, yet accepting full responsibility as her attendant, such women are natural midwives.
Without the presence and acceptance of the midwife, obstetrics becomes ag-
gressive, technological and inhumane."
      Crucial to the definition of the midwife as the person responsible for giving
care to normal childbearing women is the idea that this care consists of emotional support as well as technical skills. This central idea is developed in the
book *Spiritual Midwifery* (1980) by the American lay midwife Ina May Gaskin,
who says:

> We have found that there are laws as constant as the laws of physics, electricity or
> astronomy, whose influence on the progress of birth cannot be ignored. The mid-
> wife . . . attending births must be flexible enough to discover the way these laws
> work and learn how to work within them. Pregnant and birthing women are ele-

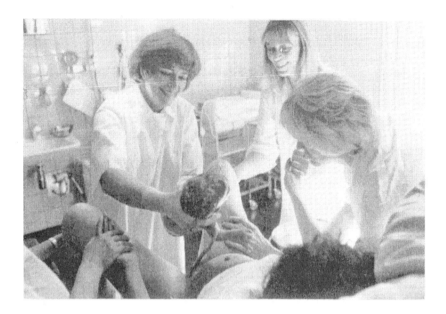

Figure 1 Danish midwife. (Photo by Jo Selsing.)

mental forces, in the same sense that gravity, thunderstorms, earthquakes and hurricanes are elemental forces. A midwife . . . needs to understand about how the energy of childbirth flows—to not know is to be like the physicist who does not understand about gravity.

A Danish midwife writes that "the midwife must know herself, so that she knows what is going on between the woman, the man and the child. It's easiest if she knows them from the beginning of the pregnancy. She needs to help the woman and the man, making sure that they have just as much help in the postpartum period as they did before and during the birth. They must have peace to get to know the baby and each other in the new situation. This situation is new with every new child that is born."

The key phrases are: to know oneself, know the family, give people space to know one another. A midwife can judge a couple's security with each other and their commitment to the child, both before and after it is born. During the labor, they do not need to be constantly told how far the birth has progressed; they are in the process, it belongs to them. They want the midwife and other helpers to join them in this. They want to receive help from them if problems develop, but they are fully aware that they themselves are closest to the child. The midwife has important work to do in the circle around the family. She can see for herself when she needs to go into this inner circle, when others should enter, and when to pull out of the circle again. She is the connection, the person who can get help from outside when necessary. There are different ways of getting such help. For example, the midwife can call someone she knows will help her in a difficult situation. Whatever she does must be best for the mother, the child, and the father.

Besides this, the midwife must be good at her work. The best tools she has are her hands, then her senses (smell, sight, and hearing). Intelligence helps, and intuition is a must.

Another midwife says, "The midwife is a servant, not a goddess. She's there to serve you and to bring her skills and knowledge, but, beyond that, it's not her business. The birth belongs to the parents."

What do parents think of midwives? These are the feelings of some parents about the midwives who have helped them:

A midwife is there to support you and help you.

Our midwife told us all the time what she was doing, and that gives you such a feeling of safety.

A midwife has no routines. . . . she is *in* the situation and responds to it individually, and that makes you feel secure.

For me, the midwife was everything. . . . She was the one I gave birth together with, she was the one I listened to. In a way, I had nothing to say myself, because my body gave me the messages I needed; I followed the needs of my body. My midwife (whom I knew) gave answers and help according to my body's needs. I *was* my body, it was she who did the physical things. . . . To give birth with a midwife I did not know already—I could not imagine that.

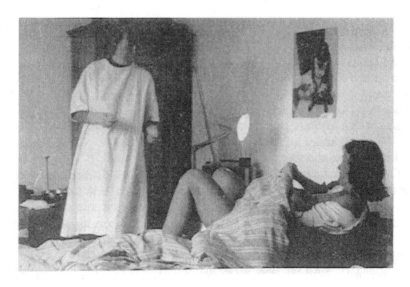

Figure 2   Danish home birth.

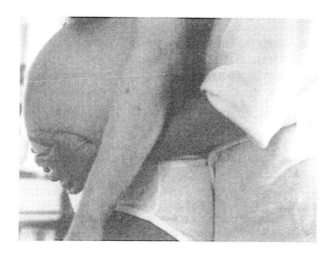

Figure 3 Midwife's hands.

These individual reactions identify key elements in the role of midwives today and in the past: personal support, continuity of care, sensitivity to the mother's needs. These values are emphasized in more systematic surveys of patient satisfaction. Looking at the North American literature on nurse-midwifery in a study for the U.S. Office of Technology Assessment, Brooks found that mothers readily identify greater ease of communication, and more "patient" control over labor and delivery, as characteristics of midwife care. Women also say that midwives keep their clients waiting for much shorter times than physicians, on average. Women having babies share with all social groups a tendency to be satisfied with the status quo, so that this fact has to be remembered when making sense of the literature on patient satisfaction. Yet what stands out is that women are more likely to feel satisfied and confident about the care given by midwives than about that given by doctors. In North America, these differences in women's attitudes are reflected in the much lower incidence of malpractice suits for nurse-midwives. A national survey in the United States in 1982 found that 5 percent of certified nurse-midwives, compared with 31 percent of obstetricians, admitted having been sued at some time (20 percent of obstetricians had been sued at least three times).

MIDWIVES ON MIDWIFERY

Elisabeth Davis, a California midwife, writes, "Midwifery is a way of life, both grueling and transformative. The continual learning on high levels has definite effects; after a year or so of practice comes the discovery that midwifery is a whole lot more than the joy of catching babies. It makes us work on all levels, either by disintegrating or integrating us." A West German midwife says, "My work means everything to me, and I hope that none of the women that I help gets the feeling she is just a number. I must help them to experience birth as the greatest, most natural experience that exists."

Midwifery can be an extremely exhausting occupation. In my (Susanne Houd) own work as a midwife during a time when I was constantly on call for home births, I wrote:

> When I work like this, I must have two kinds of readiness: one is a daily readiness; I have to be ready with everything practical. This reminds me of my own pregnancies, when everything had to be ready all the time. Now, arrangements for my children have to be 100% secure, because of my work as a midwife. When I'm home, I spend as much time together with them as possible. I can never promise anything in the future, only what I can do here and now. I feel it is very important that my children don't get allergic to births.
>
> I can't begin big projects. I have to be rested all the time. My love life suffers. It's difficult to get really involved in making love when you know the phone can ring any minute. But, interestingly, I'd thought beforehand that it would be worse. For slowly, this way of working has become a lifestyle.
>
> The other kind of readiness I experience during the births themselves is a feeling of being *there—right now—*at *that* birth *now:* time stops, and I get the feeling that my soul and my calmness is with me and we dive into timelessness together. But this doesn't always happen. Sometimes I'm impatient—I can't listen to the way the birth is going, and then I start to interfere.

I later experienced the same kind of dive into timelessness when I visited the midwives at The Farm in Tennessee, who consciously work with and around the energy of the woman giving birth.

All the midwives quoted so far work independently and mainly with home births. They work like this despite reactions from other professionals, which are often hostile, and despite the fact that their work usually means long, hard hours and little money. What about the other kinds of midwife—the ones who work within the system, in hospitals and clinics, who have scheduled time off, and get a salary every month, no matter how much or how little they do?

Anna Maxen is a midwife in a small hospital maternity unit in Denmark. The hospital is the only one on its island. There are about a hundred births a year. Three midwives handle all the antenatal visits and births. Anna lives five minutes from the hospital and has worked there for several years. She says, "I like my job very much. Because there are only the three of us midwives, we know each other very well, and the women know all of us. We also meet them in other situations, like your kids go to the same school or you meet them in the supermarket. I like that. We've pushed ourselves into the hospital clinic as well, so now the doctors think that it can't work without us. When there were fewer births, we had to find other work areas, and we had so many complaints about the doctors in the clinic, the women didn't want to go there.''

Midwife Beatrice Dana works at a university hospital in Denmark, where she has no chance of getting to know the women she delivers. This concerns her very much, and she tries to get as much out of each birth as possible, even though she says it is difficult to find the right balance. She says that she wants to be sensitive to each woman's needs, but "I don't know who she is or how she feels: she knows best herself. When she comes in to hospital, whether it's during the pregnancy or during the birth, I try to help her to decide how she wants the rest of the pregnancy or the birth to happen. She has to make up her own mind."

A midwife in the Netherlands, mainly working with home births but within the official system of care, talks about her way of working: "When I work, I use my instinct. On the whole, I treat every pregnancy individually. Categories of risk are a nuisance because, in fact, you might miss somebody who is not in one of your categories. I hate all these rules of thumb. I think midwives and other people have used them far too much anyway instead of using their clinical judgment."[1]

Sensitivity to the individual may be even more important for a midwife when she has no early opportunity of getting to know the women for whom she is providing care. One such midwife explained, "I look very hard at the woman, I think I can tell a lot about how she will deliver just by the way she looks." This midwife is tired of her job; she misses the opportunity for continuity of care. She has too much to do. She feels that she is not able to be sufficiently caring for the women, "but one has to survive . . . you can't give your soul every time." The need to work in shifts and countless deliveries of unknown women can exhaust midwives, so that their loyalty to their colleagues becomes greater than their loyalty to the women. This shows especially when a woman wants something different from the usual routine. For example, one midwife recounted this experience: "She told me that she wanted to stand up during the birth. But I thought to myself, oh no, I'm so tired, and what is everybody else going to say? I told her I thought it would be all right, and I went outside the room and told the others I was going to deal with this birth myself, as the woman didn't want anybody else in the room during her labor and birth. It was, of course, I who didn't want anybody there. It was difficult enough with myself, so I put a spiritual chair in front of the door, so to speak."

The practice of midwifery produces daily—and nightly—dilemmas of this kind. Writing about "The Night Shift" in the *Association of Radical Midwives Magazine,* Ishbel Kargar, a British midwife, describes how the tasks she is allocated on the antenatal ward provoke her to think not only about what midwifery *is,* but what it *ought* to be:

[1]The issue of risk categories is discussed in Chapter 6.

I walk upstairs, hoping that some of the women have gone home, as the night before we had a completely full ward, and as more than half of the 17 beds were occupied by postnatal mothers (a common occurrence). . . . We had been kept very busy all night. I find it rather frustrating to know that I am only able to give a fraction of the assistance most of these women need. . . .

My hopes have been realized, and of the 17 women I had left on the ward that morning there are now only half remaining. Some of the first-time mothers have gone home, too, and I feel that they are probably going to have a more restful night in their own beds, with only their own babies to disturb their sleep. It seems amazing to me that we don't hear more complaints from postnatal women about the noise of other babies. . . . The antenatal women are the ones who suffer from a mixed ward, and as they are usually admitted for "rest," it rather makes a mockery of the admission policy. . . .

Next is the medicine round, and the inevitable requests for painkillers begin. I am in constant conflict with myself, wondering how I, as a lone midwife, can reverse this mass acceptance of drug-taking as a way of life and wishing I could see more progress in the avoidance of episiotomy. There have been great reductions in these operations over the past few years, but the numbers being done are still far higher than in some units . . . and I feel that we should be looking at alternative ways of conducting labour and comparing results more than we do. . . .

Tonight I am unable to take my meal break away from the ward, as there are no midwives free to relieve me, so I make a cup of tea and sit down in the office with my sandwiches, hoping that I will be able to put my feet up for a short while, at least. Fat chance! The drip counter alarm sounds, and I spend the next ten minutes arguing with a piece of modern technology which seems to have a mind of its own. . . .

A call bell rings, and I am called to a woman who had been admitted for observation the day before, as she is a few days overdue and her blood pressure had risen slightly. Mrs B tells me she has been having contractions for about an hour, and they are now about five minutes apart. It is her third baby, and she recognizes the signs of true labour. I suggest she let me examine her; then we can decide whether she needs to go round to the labour ward yet. . . . She agrees, and we are pleasantly surprised to find that her cervix is 6 cm dilated. Her blood pressure is normal, and she doesn't want any analgesia, but opts to go to the labour ward, since her husband can then come in and be with her in labour, and she can walk around without disturbing her sleeping companions. This is when I wish we had a "Know Your Midwife"[2] scheme running, as it would have been so good to take her round to the labour ward, look after her in labour, help her to deliver her baby and then bring her back to the ward and carry on looking after them both. (p. 16)

Dissatisfaction with such conditions of practice sometimes leads to a midwife breaking away altogether. An independent midwife, Melody Weig, working in England, explains what led to her decision to do work on her own:

[2]See page 56.

I was always interested in independent midwifery, even as a pupil, and my experience in NHS [National Health Service] hospitals was enough to convince me. I met women in labor, helped them give birth and often never saw them again. . . .

Then there was the frustration of working with doctors at SHO[3] level, who, for the most part, had little experience and few specialist skills but who distrusted midwives and were taking over more and more of midwifery care. Why did all laboring women have to be clerked and periodically seen by doctors? Could a midwife not ascertain that a woman was in normal labor and call for help if necessary? Having trained with the belief that no labor is normal except in hindsight, the doctors' anxiety was soon transmitted to all around, and their willingness to interfere in what should have been normal midwifery cases led to many unnecessary interventions.

I was equally frustrated by some of my midwife colleagues, who seemed as stuck in their ways as the doctors. Why so many episiotomies, routine admission procedures of shaves and enemas, and routine observations in labor? No labor is routine; why try to make it so? . . . My attempts to change even small things seemed to fall on deaf ears.

I left because numerous incidents, procedures, and policies served only to undermine my midwifery skills and confidence, mystify the women they were meant to help, and turn the birth experience into a medically controlled "procedure."

I am all for modern obstetrics, but in the true meaning of the word: that it be practiced scientifically, that all interventions be of proven value, that the value outweigh the risks in each case, and that we wait and work with the process in a supportive and trusting rather than an interfering and worrying way.

Melody Weig's point about the desirability of practicing scientific obstetrics is an extremely important one for midwives today; we come back to it later.

All these midwives work in the developed part of Europe, but the constraints on the midwife's autonomy can be similar in other countries. A midwife from a less developed country describes her working history: "I've worked in a state hospital with many deliveries every day. In a way, I liked it because nobody, I mean no doctors, came and took over—I could do as I wanted. But in another way it was awful; sometimes you deliver six or seven babies in eight hours. It's impossible to get any kind of personal contact with the women. Mind you, most of them just want to get it over and done with."

A midwife in Morocco, working in a "birth house," says she has been here for twenty-five years. She has nothing to do with the women in pregnancy, meeting them for the first time when they're in labor, but she feels this is all right because "I'm here most of the time; I like being a midwife here; everybody in the neighborhood knows me."

Midwives have rarely revealed to others what it is like to be a midwife. In

[3]Senior house officer, below consultant and registrar level.

the past, they have seldom talked to each other about it. Being a midwife can be a very lonely business. In part, this is because of the importance of birth—the fact that it is a human event of tremendous importance to the individual, the family, and the community. In part, it is because of the way birth has been divided up among different professional groups, put in institutions, and rendered increasingly a medical and technological process. Wherever they work in the developed world, midwives have to find their way around complex bureaucratic and professional rules, and they must negotiate their own authentic space in the midst of confusing professional antagonisms and with continual regard for the needs of the women and families with whom they are working.

HOW MANY MIDWIVES?

It is surprisingly difficult to get correct and up-to-date information on midwives in Europe. Women who have trained as midwives may not be active in midwifery, or they may be working as nurses and thus registered in the statistics as nurses rather than as midwives. In some countries where midwives are also nurses, another cause of statistical invisibility is that it may be cheaper to belong to nursing associations than midwifery associations. In some places, midwifery is actually defined as a specialty of nursing, which makes the correct figure for the number of active midwives impossible to come by. One way of looking at the numbers of midwives in practice is in relation to the population of the country. There is significant variation here, as Table 1 shows. The figures in this table range from 129.5 midwives per 100,000 population in the Soviet Union to only 11.4 per 100,000 in Ireland. Changes over time move in both directions, with some countries increasing and some decreasing their midwife-to-population ratio. In general, however, despite these variations, it is true to say that for two decades the number and density of midwives have been declining all over Europe.

The reasons behind changes in the midwifery labor force are as complex as those behind the rise and fall of any occupational group. Shifting birth rates and other changes in the position of women, tightened legislation, the move toward institutional birth, increased use of technology—these are some factors. Statistics themselves are influenced by social forces. For example, in England between the late 1970s and the mid-1980s, there was an apparently large increase in the numbers of nursing and midwifery staff, but about half of this "increase" was due to a changed definition of the working week, which inflated the statistics, while the number of people working remained the same.

In a few countries, special efforts have been made to find out how many midwives actually work as midwives. In Norway, for example, it was found that only 700 out of 1700 trained midwives actually worked as midwives. The rest either were not using their training or were working as nurses. In a survey reported by Josephine Golden in the United Kingdom, recently qualified mid-

Table 1 Midwives per 100,000 Population in Selected
European Countries

Country	Number per 100,000 population[a]	Annual percentage change since early 1970s
Belgium	18.3	−4.9
Czechoslovakia	44.9	+0.6
Denmark	14.0	+6.2
Finland	17.1	−3.4
France	16.8	+1.1
Greece	34.5	+7.3
Hungary	25.7	+3.5
Ireland	11.4	−9.8
Italy	29.1	−1.5
Switzerland	22.4	−1.9
Turkey	31.2	−1.2
U.S.S.R.	129.5	+1.1
United Kingdom	36.9	−0.4
Yugoslavia	35.2	+3.3

[a]Varies by country from 1980–84. In France and Greece, 1977.
Source: WHO (1986, unpublished data).

wives were asked their career intentions. More than two thirds did not intend to make a career in midwifery; one in ten, even so short a time (a matter of months) after qualifying, did not intend to practice at all. A number of studies conducted in this century have shown that fewer than 40 percent of qualifying midwives in the United Kingdom train because they want to practice: more than half use midwifery to further their nursing careers. Dissatisfaction with conditions of service and job prospects in midwifery are another reason for a lack of intention to use a midwifery training. One in four of a group of midwives qualifying in England in 1983 gave these as reasons why they did not intend to work as midwives.

WHERE DO MIDWIVES WORK?

Midwives work in hospitals, homes, and clinics. They are employed by the government, either centrally or locally. They work independently, either supported by the government or totally outside the system. However, to map out exactly where midwives work from existing data obtainable from international sources is difficult.

In the Netherlands in 1984, the number of practicing midwives was 860; of these, 16 percent were employed by hospitals and 69 percent worked independently, two thirds of these in solo practices. Forty-two percent of all deliveries

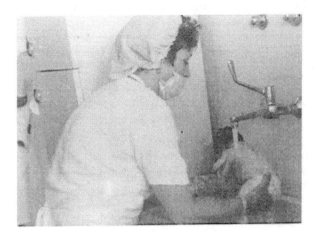

Figure 4   Midwife and baby in hospital.

that year were attended by midwives. Figure 6 gives an idea of the changes in the numbers of Dutch midwives since 1970 in relation to the two other main professional groups concerned with childbirth: general practitioners and obstetrician-gynecologists. The latter group is clearly profiting in terms of rapidly increased numbers.

In Italy, about six hundred new midwives are now licensed every year. In 1982, 69 percent of practicing midwives worked in the national health care system—half in hospitals, where they attended almost all the births, and the other half in the community, either supervised by local health authorities and

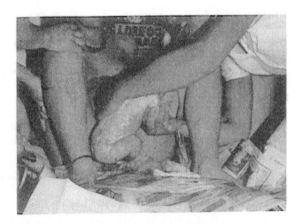

Figure 5   Midwife and baby at home.

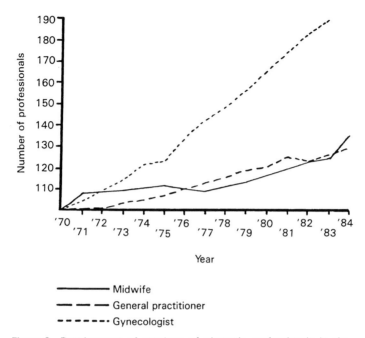

——————— Midwife

— — — General practitioner

- - - - - - Gynecologist

Figure 6 Development of numbers of obstetric professionals in the Netherlands since 1970. (From van Daalen, 1988, with data from Hessing-Wagner, 1985.)

working fairly independently or in family health practices (a recent development in Italy). Private hospitals employed 4 percent of all midwives, and 27 percent either worked in private practice or were retired (it is impossible to tell from the statistics whether a midwife is retired or not, since there is no age limit for a midwife in Italy).

As will be seen in the rest of this book, the theme of the midwife's competition with the obstetrician-gynecologist for the care and control of childbearing women is absolutely central to the situation of midwives in Europe today. The 1985 WHO report, *Having a Baby in Europe*, had this to say:

Over the last 50 years, there has been a gradual decrease in the role of the midwife in providing care to pregnant women in the official services. Today, in most countries of the European Region, the visits to official services by women during pregnancy are divided between midwives and physicians. The midwife is the sole provider during pregnancy only in those areas where there are shortages of physicians. There are, however, other countries or areas where no midwives provide care during pregnancy, only physicians.

There are also changes in the role of physicians in the officially sanctioned services for pregnant women. The most prevalent trend is an increasing role for

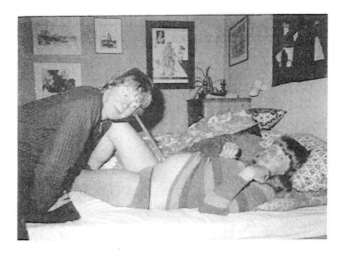

Figure 7 Styles of care-giving: the midwife at home.

obstetricians, even with uncomplicated pregnancies, with a decreased use of general practitioners. . . .

The way in which health personnel assist women during birth is at present changing considerably. In most countries, obstetricians are now in charge of most or all births. In some countries, midwives remain in charge of uncomplicated births, referring any complications to the physician, while in a few countries, midwives are in charge of all births, uncomplicated and complicated, relinquishing

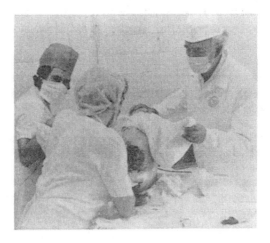

Figure 8 Part of the "team."

responsibility only for Caesarean section. . . . As births move into big hospitals, physicians in training participate more in births. The overall trend, therefore, is for physicians more and more to take responsibility for all births. As a result, midwives find themselves more and more becoming physicians' assistants. This is a significant trend, since midwives (at least in the past) and physicians have had, in general, quite different styles of care during birth.

In other words, midwives and obstetricians are not interchangeable as providers of care for childbearing women. They have different histories, which help to account for their different styles of care. Thus, before looking at what midwives actually do in caring for childbearing women today, it is necessary to look at the emergence of the profession from its beginnings in the informal care given by women to one another during this both ordinary and extraordinary event called "having a baby."

Midwives in History

The origins of the term *midwife* speak to, and about, the current crisis in midwifery: what kind of person should a midwife be, and what should she do? In English, *midwife* means "a woman who is with the mother at birth." To use the word *midwife* is thus to refer to a long tradition of alliance between the women giving birth and the women attending them. As a matter of fact, the term *obstetric* originally carried the same meaning; in the mid-eighteenth century, the Latin word *obstetrix* began to be used to refer to "a woman who is present to receive the child."

Other languages express the alliance between midwives and mothers in different ways. In Danish, the word for midwife (*jordmor*) means, literally, "earth mother." In the old days, a birth took place on the ground, and the midwife was there to lift the child from the ground. She was also called "earth mother" because it was widely believed that, in order to practice as a midwife, a woman should be a mother herself.

How did the role of midwife emerge, acquire a name, and become accepted in society? At what point did the term *obstetric* acquire its modern meaning of a male-dominated medical profession distinct in important ways from the traditional practice of midwifery? How have childbearing women accommodated themselves to, or protested against, these profound changes in the care available to them at a very important time in their lives? This chapter takes what is necessarily a quick look at some of these important historical issues.

OLD WIVES' TALES: WOMEN AS HEALERS AND MIDWIVES

The deliverers of babies throughout human history have been women, and so have their principal attendants. Even today, it has been estimated that some 80 percent of all births in the world are attended by midwives of one kind or another. The association between midwives and women is even more extensive than this would indicate.

Before the rise of the modern medical profession, women in most countries performed most of the healing and caring work that needed to be done. This is still true today. As part of their normal domestic role, women provide more health care than all the world's health services put together. The most important health care unit is the household, not the hospital. Within the household, women in all countries, at all stages of economic development, undertake most of the work needed for the maintenance of people's health and the serving of their daily needs. In particular, the care of children and elderly or disabled dependents is labeled women's work. As official health services develop, women also contribute the major part of the labor required for these, although they are underrepresented among doctors and overrepresented among nurses, clerical workers, cleaners, and lower grade medical-service specialities.

The historical relationship between women and midwives is thus part of the jigsaw puzzle of women's past and present health care work. One problem with this work, and with this perspective, is that it is not a part of the official version of history. Most health care histories concentrate on the political and economic superstructure and on phenomena, such as professionalization, that chiefly involve the male work force. Most such histories take the division of labor between men and women for granted, which means that they tend to allocate to women an invisible and inferior domestic role. Women become visible only in the occasional historical moments during which they protest the role they have traditionally been given.

Old wife is one term for a traditional woman healer and midwife. Others are *good woman, cunning woman* (*cunning* meaning "knowing more than others"), or *wisewoman* (the French word for midwife is still *sage-femme*). Such women were the main providers of health and midwifery care in preindustrial Europe and colonial North America. They were, indeed, the only medical and obstetric practitioners available to a community living in constant poverty and disease. During this period, health care and attendance at childbirth were regarded in all social groups as an important part of women's role within the family and the household. For example, one eighteenth-century English aristo-crat wrote to his wife telling her to "give the child no phisick but such as midwives and old women . . . do prescribe; for assure yourself they by experi-ence know better than any physition how to treat such infants."

The care of infants and of women in childbirth was something women would learn by experience, so experience and age were the main qualifications for acceptance as a community healer and midwife. Figure 9 shows an early-fifteenth-century birth room scene; at this time female midwifery was common in all social classes in Europe. Midwives were expected to be mature married women with children of their own, and skills were passed from mother to daughter. In rural England in the seventeenth century, according to A. Clark, "It was customary, when travail began, to send for all the neighbours who were responsible women, partly with the object of securing enough witnesses to the child's birth, partly because it was important to spread the understanding of midwifery as widely as possible because any woman might be called upon to render assistance in an emergency."

This, incidentally, is the origin of the word *gossip,* which, like *old wives* (in the phrase *old wives' tales*), is now used only in a derogatory sense. A gossip was originally a woman called to witness a childbirth. Old wives' tales were originally the knowledge relating to the treatment of illness possessed by traditional women healers. Both terms are now used to refer disparagingly to attributes of modern women. Women today may have gained important legal and social rights, but they have also sustained some losses in stature as com-pared with their preindustrial counterparts.

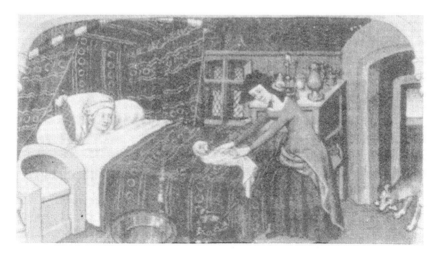

Figure 9   A birth room scene, fifteenth century.

The opposite of old wives' tales is young doctors' tales. The development of modern medical knowledge has caused the latter to be defined as healing strategies superior to the empirical methods for treating both illness and reproduction that were practiced by old wives. However, the questioning spirit provoked by feminism and the alternative health movements of the last fifteen to twenty years have shown both the mythology of much modern "scientific medicine" and the inherent scientific wisdom of some of the old wives' practices.

We now know that such practices as induction of labor, predelivery shaving and enemas, electronic fetal heart rate monitoring in labor, and prenatal ultrasound scanning have no scientific basis as routine practices—that is, their routine use does not guarantee better survival or health for mother or child. Conversely, the practices of traditional women healers and midwives were often scientifically effective. For example, when old wives used to start labor with five, seven, or nine black grains growing on rye in wet, cold weather, they were employing a potent modern drug, ergot. When male obstetricians discovered this and used ergot in their own practices, they applied it so overenthusiastically that they must have caused at least as much harm as they prevented.

Very many compounds and treatments used by wisewomen and other community healers have subsequently been shown to have a scientific basis. A review in 1981 by Antonio Scarpa of the Institute of Ethnomedicine in Italy revealed that 230 plants regarded traditionally as having therapeutic value had been proved to contain an active therapeutic ingredient, according to the methods of modern scientific medicine. Inoculation against smallpox, for example, was originally a folk remedy practiced by midwives and other healers. It was a true sign of the times when, in the 1840s in England, the government banned inoculation because the medical profession declared it dangerous, and the Catholic Church conspired with this verdict by defining it as sinful.

In her book *Old Wives' Tales*, Mary Chamberlain lists twenty-nine pharmaceutical compounds that were part of the practices of women healers and midwives in the past and are still listed in the British Pharmaceutical Codex today. Nine others disappeared only recently from the official list. Some continue to be approved for use in other countries; French and Spanish doctors, for instance, still make official use of garlic.

It was characteristic of the practice of old wives that they did not separate the use of plants and herbs from that of "ritual" charms and incantations. The following treatment for whooping cough comes from a nineteenth-century collection of folk remedies: "Pass the child nine times under and over a donkey three years old. Then take three spoonfuls of milk drawn from one teat of one animal and three hairs cut from its back, and three hairs cut from its belly. Place the hairs in the milk and let it stand for three hours. Then give it to the child in three doses." An unpleasant-sounding strategy, this nonetheless would have been likely to induce vomiting and thus provide temporary relief.

Significantly, Mary Chamberlain (1981) took her excursion into the annals

of unofficial history (*Old wives tales: Their history, remedies, and spells*) because she herself is the great-granddaughter of an "old wife": "They called my
great-grandmother the 'Angel of Alsace Street'. If anyone was in labour, she
would be there with her basins and rags delivering the babies and attending the
mothers. If anyone was sick, the first person they would fly to was old
grandma. When neighbours died, she laid them out. She took care of her local
community in birth and death, and for much of the period in between. . . . My
great-grandmother had 16 children, and this was deemed sufficient qualification
[for her role]."

About the same time, in the early twentieth century, in an English village
(Grey, 1977):

> The people seemed to depend in maternity cases upon the elder and more experi-
> enced of the married women just round about. There were some few of the cottag-
> ers who could afford to engage a doctor on these occasions and did so, but the
> majority of the women of the labouring class . . . would arrange for one or the
> other of the experienced neighbours to attend her at these times. . . . Several of the
> elder of the cottage women were very clever and efficient midwives; in fact, there
> were some few quite famed in the neighbourhood for their ability and efficiency, so
> much so, that they were often engaged by people of considerable means. . . . They
> would go to the cottage each morning and night for some little time after the birth,
> to attend to mother and child, wash, change, and put them comfortable.

Although this form of integrated care has largely disappeared in industrialized countries, it is, of course, still common in the Third World. In Nigeria, for
example, 80 percent of the population live in rural areas and have access only to
traditional healers. There are seven different categories of such healers, of
whom traditional birth attendants are one. These are usually elderly women
and, as with all such traditional healers, a recognized period and system of
training precedes independent practice. A survey by Oyebola (1980) of traditional healers among the Yoruba of Nigeria showed that "the process of training
is one of apprenticeship of the would-be trainee to an established practitioner.
Generally, there are no rigid preconditions for admission into the course. . . .
The only condition for rejection of training as a traditional healer is if the
would-be apprentice is discovered to be incompetent in coping with the training
programme."

During the process of development, some countries incorporate traditional
healers into the official system of care provision. In the village of Gizera,
Somalia, midwife Batula Hassan began to help local women to deliver their
babies at the age of eleven. Her grandmother was the village midwife, and she
began by taking Batula along to cut the cord and hold the baby. When Somalia's
nationwide literacy campaign was launched in 1973, Batula learned to read and
then took a four-month government-organized course on basic hygiene and

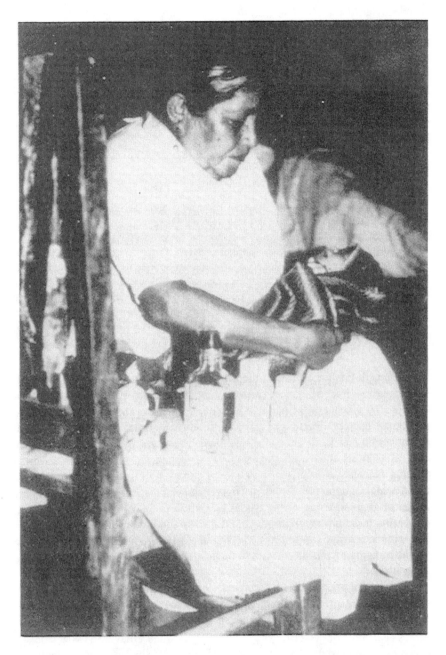

Figure 10   A Guatemalan traditional midwife with swaddled newborn child; beside her is the candle used to cauterize the end of the umbilical cord and alcohol to dress it.

health care. By the late 1970s, she rarely had fewer than ten deliveries a month, which sometimes involved nomadic families and entailed spending several days away from home.

In 1978, when the World Health Organization (WHO) goal of health for all by the year 2000 was formulated in Alma-Ata, U.S.S.R., the traditional midwife was recognized as being an important ally in the expansion of primary health care. Renamed by WHO the traditional birth attendant (TBA), she had already been defined as "a person (usually a woman) who assists the mother at childbirth and who initially acquired her skills delivering babies by herself or by working with other TBAs." A British missionary midwife working in Sudan was the first to set up a training program for TBAs in 1921. In 1985, the governments of at least twenty-three Third World countries had given official recognition to TBAs. Many others were in the process of doing so and of setting up training programs for them.

Some countries have trained primary health workers in medical and surgical procedures that, in the West, would be seen as quite beyond their expertise. In northwestern Zaire, for example, nurses have been trained to carry out Caesarean sections, laparotomies, and hysterectomies in a successful effort to reduce the high rate of maternal deaths.

This profile of the typical TBA was included in a survey of TBAs' practices by E. Leedam, in the *International Journal of Obstetrics and Gynecology,* published in 1985:

> The TBA is usually an older woman, almost always past menopause, and has borne one or more children herself. She lives in the community in which she practises. She operates in a relatively restricted zone, limited to her own village and sometimes those adjacent. Her role includes everything connected with the conduct of childbirth. . . . The TBA is often an accomplished herbalist, whose knowledge and use of herbs, roots and barks can be quite extensive. . . . To common problems she works out solutions within a framework of values and beliefs shared with her client. She participates in the same cycle of cultural activity and is a recognized member of the same social universe. (p. 250)

Table 2 shows how important the health care work of this group is in relation to that of other health professionals in poor communities.

Even in the developed world, the institution of traditional midwifery survives. Turning to the United States, for example, in North Carolina in the 1930s, some two thirds of nonwhite deliveries were attended by midwives at home. Many of these midwives were traditional "granny midwives": 15 percent of them were seventy years old or more. In addition, according to J. B. Litoff's history of American midwives, they were women "of vast personal experience of childbirth." Only 23 percent had borne fewer than seven children of their own. Figure 11 shows a British "granny midwife" earlier in the cen-

Table 2   Physicians, Nurses, and TBAs per 10,000 Population in Six Countries

Country	Year	Physicians	Nurses	TBAs
Afghanistan	1973	0.4	0.2	12.8
Guatemala	1976	3.2	2.4	31.3
Haiti	1973	1.3	1.1	20.4
Indonesia	1973	0.5	0.6	27.8
Nicaragua	1974	5.9	11.1	21.3
Thailand	1975	1.3	3.1	7.1

Source: Leedam, 1985.

tury, compared to the newer licensed and regulated version holding her bicycle, symbol of women's independence.

Whether or not the official system takes over traditional healing and midwifery, the traditional system is likely to be maintained by popular belief and custom, at least for a while. One example of this from a different field is a 1985 survey of Tanzanians with cancer, by C. A. Alexander, which found that 49 percent of the women and 41 percent of the men attending a hospital for radiation treatment had previously consulted traditional healers. The most common cancer thus treated was cancer of the cervix. Worldwide, it has been estimated that 75–80 percent of the population today uses traditional "prescientific" health treatments.

LOSING GROUND: THE MEDICAL AND OBSTETRICAL TAKEOVERS

Two periods of transition lie between this situation and the current one in industrialized countries in which midwives are threatened and where women's health care role has been buried in the "hidden health care system." The first was the emergence of professionalized medicine and the exclusion of women from it (a position that they have subsequently had to fight to reverse). During this first period of transition, formal training for midwives was started, and their professional relationship with doctors began to be defined and codified—to the midwives' increasing disadvantage. The second period of transition, which merges with the first, takes the form of the colonization of midwifery by a new medical speciality—obstetrics.

These historical processes have taken different forms in different countries. Most notably, what happened in North America was in contrast to developments in Europe: the North American midwife was successfully banished from the obstetrical scene, while midwifery never disappeared from Europe. The masculinization of medicine and the erosion of the midwife's autonomy are, however, common international themes.

Witches and Doctors

Understanding why and how these transitions occurred is not an easy task. One factor that stands out is the associations among the terms *woman, witch, midwife,* and *wisewoman.*

"At this time," wrote one Englishman in 1584, "It is indifferent to say in the English tongue 'she is a witch' or 'she is a wisewoman'." An Act of Parliament in 1511 was directed at the "great multitude of ignorant persons," among whom were "common artificers, as smythes, weavers and women,"

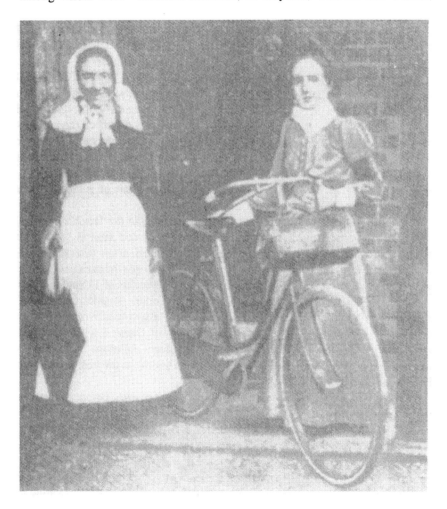

Figure 11 The Midwives Act of 1902 in England brought change to the old "gianny midwife" (left) with the arrival of the better trained licensed midwife (right).

who "took upon themselves great cures and thinges of great difficultie in which they partly use sorcery, and witchcrafte." There is abundant evidence that in medieval Europe some practicing midwife-healers were accused and convicted of witchcraft. Witch hunts were a widespread phenomenon in Europe between the fourteenth and seventeenth centuries. Most of those convicted were women, because most healers were women and the term *witch* was much more likely to be attached to a woman than a man. In the Salem witch trials in seventeenth-century New England, 74 percent of accused witches were women. The typical witch was a married or widowed woman aged between forty-one and sixty years, and the males accused of witchcraft tended to be the children or husbands of female witches. It is not surprising to find that most would-be doctors disapproved of lay female healers. Established religion, of course, disapproved of witchcraft, too; the suppression of witchcraft and popular beliefs in magic was a necessary step in the establishment of an official state religion.

One reason why both the state and the church were opposed to female midwifery was that there were no external controls on midwives' activities. No body of legislation controlled what midwives did or where, with whom, and how they worked. Moreover, it was plain that midwives did more than deliver babies. To respond to the needs of women in the community, the midwife-healer had to provide contraceptive advice, help in procuring abortion, and remedies for infertility. Female midwives were thus part of a female-controlled reproductive care system. It was precisely this that posed so much of a threat to the church, the state, and the emerging medical profession.

The charge that midwives, through their alliance with the Devil, destroyed infants before or shortly after birth begins to be recorded around 1460. The famous European witch-hunting manual *Malleus maleficarum* (literally *Hammer of Witches*, produced in a pocket-size edition that witch-hunters could carry with them at all times) contains many elaborate accusations of infanticide. For example: "We must not omit to mention the injuries done to children by witch midwives, first by killing them, and secondly by blasphemously offering them to devils . . . in the diocese of Basel at the town of Dana, a witch who was burned confessed that she had killed more than forty children, by sticking a needle through the crown of their heads into their brains, as they came out from the womb" (Kramer & Sprenger, 1971).

Some such accusations were founded on the fact that, before the era of modern contraceptive methods, induced abortion was a major means of fertility control. The phenomenon of witchcraft has attracted a lot of attention from historians, who have come up with various theories to explain it. Almost by definition, perhaps, the accusation of witchcraft is synonymous with hostility to women and women's real or imagined power. Certainly, a tone of antagonism toward women is marked, not only in much of the historical evidence relating to witchcraft but also in the pronouncements of twentieth-century medical experts. *A Textbook of the Science and Art of Obstetrics* written by H. J. Garrigues

(1902) around the turn of the century declared, in tones reminiscent of the *Malleus maleficarum,* that:

> midwives do harm not only through their lack of obstetric knowledge, their neglect of antiseptic precautions, and their tendency to conceal undesirable features, but most of them are the most inveterate quacks. First of all they treat disturbances occurring during the puerpery, late gynaecological diseases, then diseases of children, and finally they are consulted in regard to almost everything. They never acknowledge their ignorance, and are always ready to give advice . . . their thinly veiled advertisements in the newspapers show them to be willing abortionists; and, since they have the right to give certificates of stillbirth, who knows whether or not an infant's death is due to natural causes or to criminal manipulations?

Underlying these deeply held suspicions is another fascinating dimension of social attitudes to women and women's traditional healing/midwifery role. Midwives and women have been felt to be threatening because of their sexual identities. Men (particularly witch-hunters) complained of women's insatiable sexual lust: "All witchcraft comes from carnal lust, which is in women insatiable . . . these women satisfy their filthy lusts not only in themselves, but even in the mighty ones of the age, of whatever state and condition, causing by all sorts of witchcraft the death of their souls through the excessive infatuation of carnal love" (Kramer & Sprenger, 1971). According to the *Malleus maleficarum,* women's sexual appetites drove them to have congress with the Devil and to use their work as midwives for this purpose!

The early control of midwives was the responsibility of the church, not the state. In medieval witch trials, the male doctor was the expert summoned by the church; at this time, university-trained physicians were themselves not supposed to practice except with the advice of a priest. Until the thirteenth century, medical practice was open to all, and the only formal qualification available was a license gained from a university education. However, the problem for women healers was that, in most countries, they were barred from the universities, and from the thirteenth century onward medical guilds began to close their doors to those without a university license. By the sixteenth century, the three orders of medical practitioners—physicians, surgeons, and apothecaries—were organizing themselves into corporations with some licensing authority.

These developments helped to suppress women healers and midwives by creating a hierarchy of practice: university-trained male practitioners for the upper classes and empirically trained female practitioners for the working classes. The relationship between these two groups was not always one of opposition: Nicholas Tynchewyke, the first lecturer in medicine at Oxford in the early fourteenth century, once heard a rumor of an effective remedy for jaundice and rode forty miles to obtain this from an old woman who had already cured many people with it.

Furthermore, not everyone was taken in by the heavily theoretical new academic medicine. The Doctor of Physic in Chaucer's *Canterbury Tales* is some guide to the status and mannerisms of these early, often pretentious, medical men. Chaucer paints the Doctor as an obnoxious charlatan who "knew the cause of everich maladye": "knew" in the sense of being able to fit it to a system of explanations that had never been tested empirically and, in fact, bore little relation to the real world of human bodies.

Almost as soon as medicine began to organize itself into a profession in the modern sense, the fate of midwives became a major issue. Should midwives be trained or not? It so, what sort of training should they have? What were the demarcation lines between midwifery and medicine? A sign of the potential attractiveness of training was the interim remedy of medical sponsorship. A local newspaper in the state of Delaware carried the following advertisement in 1789: "Grace Mulligan takes this opportunity to inform the public that she has been solicited to come to Wilmington to practise Midwifery; she has had the advantage of the instructions . . . of Dr. Shippen in Philadelphia better than a year and comes recommended by him in the most flattering terms." Whether Dr. Shippen in fact improved Grace Mulligan's midwifery (or vice versa) is, of course, unknown.

Midwives and Obstetricians

The second transition bringing midwifery into its full-blown contemporary crisis was the rise of the specialty of obstetrics. Until late in the nineteenth century, the medical profession was very interested in controlling healing, but not particularly interested in taking over the midwife's work. Childbirth was "women's business." It was also not a pleasant business to meddle with—an attitude found in many cultures studied by anthropologists, where reproduction is regarded as in some way polluting to society, so that it has to be contained in some geographical or metaphorical enclosure beyond the ordinary routines of social life.

Sometime around the end of the nineteenth century, this attitude changed, and the medical profession began to accept and argue that obstetrical work was a proper part of their domain. There had, of course, been male midwives before this, but they had had the status of barber-surgeons and were not highly regarded by other branches of medicine. By the mid-nineteenth century, the upper social classes in North America and in parts of Europe had begun to turn away from traditional midwives for care during childbirth, relying on doctors instead. This development did not occur without protest. Some people said that the attendance of men in childbirth was automatically offensive to women's modesty and so, partly for that reason, the medical results were not likely to be particularly good either. The early "man-midwives" worked in the dark or under a sheet "in the interests of decency" (Figure 12), which must have made

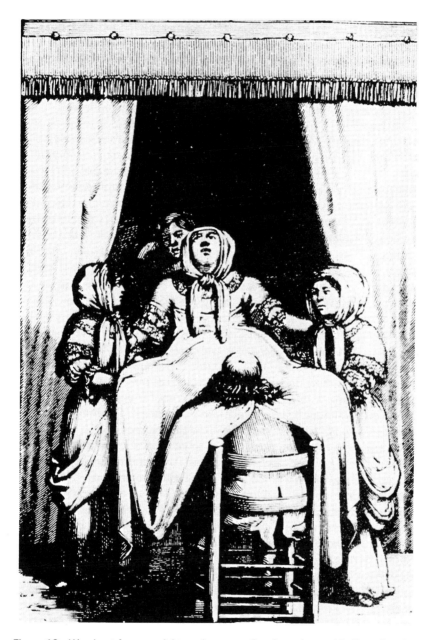

Figure 12 Wood-cut from an eighteenth-century Dutch work on midwifery showing a man-midwife attending a delivery; to maintain privacy, he has the end of the bed-sheet pinned around his neck. (From S. Janson, *Korte en Bondige verhandeling, van de voortteelingen't Kinderbaren,* Amsterdam, 1711.)

skilled attendance difficult. Some women clearly preferred to suffer in silence rather than consult a doctor. While some doctors deplored this state of affairs, others, strangely, were prepared to praise it as evidence of women's high moral tone. Such men did not want their own wives to be inspected by other men—an argument resurrected in the mid-1970s by a prominent obstetrician in the London *Times*, who said that "the husband would in most cases find difficulty in accepting another man as the primary support for his wife in labour."

Yet the real challenge was still to come. As William Arney puts it in his *Power and the Profession of Obstetrics,* "the profession of obstetrics did not result from technological imperatives or the accumulation of scientific advances. It was a strategic success." Both in North America and Europe, the triumph of obstetricians over midwives as controllers of birth represented the ascendancy of men over women, but the belief that men ought to control birth was never an overt part of the struggle. Instead, a number of more subtle (or more basic) arguments came into operation, which made control of childbirth an attractive prospect. First, doctors needed patients, and midwifery gave men an important entrée to general practice: a successful delivery meant a grateful woman and a household full of potential clients. Second, there was money to be made from delivering babies. One reason for the earlier and more complete decline of midwifery in North America was the overabundance of doctors there in the last half of the nineteenth century. Male doctors and would-be obstetricians were far too busy competing with one another for business to allow women to stake any serious claim. Third, men controlled hospitals and they needed birthing women in hospitals as teaching subjects for medical students. Fourth, and most significantly, a new definition of pregnancy and childbirth was evolving within obstetrics, which was eventually to undermine the whole rationale midwives had for attending women in childbirth.

Birth for women had always been a moral crisis, an event to be passed through and survived, a sign of character and strength. Possessing this quality, it had nevertheless been a normal part of life and of womanhood. Midwives, in helping mothers through childbirth, took the view that they were aiding and abetting nature rather than disturbing it. When obstetricians started to claim a right to decide how, where, and when childbirth happened, they needed to take the opposing view: that there was nothing normal about childbirth at all. Indeed, its "normality" consisted in its potential pathology. At any moment, and quite without warning, anything might go wrong in any pregnancy, labor, and delivery, and the presence of the obstetrical expert was needed to step in and put everything right again. Logically, this meant continual monitoring and surveillance, for the expert had to have the pregnant woman under his eyes all the time, in order to step in at the right moment.

In this contest between obstetricians and midwives, the view has been expressed again and again that the "normality" of pregnancy and childbirth is a dangerous fallacy. Critics of this view in North America in the early twentieth century amused themselves by making the extremely relevant point that many women pushed their babies out while their doctors were scrubbing up for a Caesarean. However, this sort of evidence did not matter; the only evidence that mattered was that which tended to support the argument. In 1902, a textbook of obstetrics observed that "compared with men, women have done very little for the advancement of the obstetric art" and decided that only physicians understood the principles of clean midwifery, whereas "midwives . . . are as unwilling as they are incompetent to apply them." At this time, untrained midwives delivered about half of all the babies born in New York. The author of the book, a Dr. Henry Garrigues, went on to say that mortality in births attended by midwives was twice that in doctor-attended lying-in institutions: "The pure, the healthy, the rich are apt to lose their lives by giving birth to a child in their luxurious homes, while the dissolute, those whose constitutions are undermined by disease, overwork and care, those who are struggling with poverty for mere existence, are nearly sure of leaving the hospital in a better condition than they entered it."

A few years later, another North American doctor described his vision of the midwife in New York City: "She usually goes to the scene of the labor in the ordinary dirty clothes that she has been wearing doing her household work, taking with her a satchel containing a handful of absorbent cotton and a bottle of bichloride tablets or carbolic acid, with a few strings of soiled tape for tying off the cord."

The accusation of midwife incompetence was clear, and it was made repeatedly, especially in the American medical literature. Examination of the evidence, however, has since suggested that, on the contrary and compared with the standard of obstetrics prevailing at the time, midwifery was safe. Table 3 shows some of these data for the city of Newark, New Jersey, in 1915–16. A comparison of physician-attended and midwife-attended births definitely favors midwife care, although the comparison is necessarily a crude one, making no allowance for the distribution of complicated cases between the two professional groups.

Table 3   Neonatal and Infant Mortality by Birth Attendant, In Newark, New Jersey, 1915–16

Attendant	Live births	Neonatal mortality rate[a]	Infant mortality rate[b]
Physician	11,400	43	80
Midwife	10,996	25	71

[a]Deaths per 1000 live births, significant at $p < .0005$.
[b]Deaths per 1000 live births, significant at $p < .01$.
Source: Devitt, 1979.

In pointing out the existence of social class differences in the risks of childbirth to mother and baby, Dr. Garrigues was spotting an important phenomenon. But whatever class of women went into the hospital in the late nineteenth and early twentieth centuries—whether it was the poor, who thereby could secure free care, or the rich, who thought doctor-attended childbirth a fashionable necessity—these women exposed themselves to the extra risks of hospitalization. In the era before antibiotics, sulfonamides, and efficient blood transfusion techniques, to enter the hospital to have a baby was a risk in itself. The real point was, and is, that if midwives were to be recognized as effective and safe, there would be little need for obstetricians.

To obtain clients, the early obstetricians not only had to argue the inherent pathology of pregnancy and the incompetence of midwives, but also had to appear to offer superior expertise. This expertise took the form of technology, beginning with the use by male midwives of obstetric forceps in the seventeenth century. Whether the early use of forceps saved lives, we do not know; such techniques are, on the whole, likely to have the effect of transferring mortality from one column to another—that is, they save some lives but also cause some deaths that would otherwise not have happened. It is certain that, in the early maternity hospitals, any intervention, such as the use of forceps, carried a high risk of infection, for doctors took a long time to agree with the famous Dr. Semmelweiss that gentlemen could possibly have dirty hands and thus spread infection among childbearing women. Incidentally, the original observations about the causes of puerperal fever came from a comparison of death rates among mothers attended by medical students with those among women attended by midwives. The medical students had death rates about three times as high as those of the midwives. Thus, Dr. Semmelweiss was able to argue that medical students were probably doing something dangerous (and midwives were probably doing something safe).

The 1920s and 1930s were critical years for obstetricians in many countries. During these years, they succeeded in establishing themselves organizationally as a specialist group. By the 1950s, obstetrics had discovered the fetus, and over this whole period an army of new child care experts arrived on the scene to tell mothers how to bear and bring up their children. The medical specialty to pediatrics rests some of its own professionalization on this basis. Like obstetrics, pediatrics has stolen some traditional components of midwifery, called them something else, and then defined the proper role of midwives as basically nursing. (See Figure 13.) Not only childbearing but also motherhood has been medicalized, so that any "good mother" loses her title if she fails to seek out and take professional advice. Once consulting the experts becomes a mark of morality, setting up and using alternative forms of care becomes a sign of rebellion, challenging both the doctors and the conventions of women's role in society.

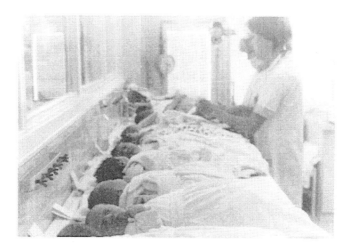

Figure 13   Nurses of newborn babies in Hungary, 1986.

HISTORY LESSONS?

Certain themes of continued contemporary interest are apparent even from this hasty journey through midwifery's past. First, the care provided by female midwives to women having babies is part of an ancient tradition of female health care. Second, the charge of incompetence as made by obstetricians against midwives and the insistence that pregnancy is essentially an illness and childbirth a time of intrinsic danger are key elements in the professional superiority that obstetricians have negotiated for themselves. Third, there is indeed a tradition of doctors and midwives having different styles of care for women in childbirth; obstetrical practice has been influenced from the beginning by the drive toward intervention (Figure 14). Finally, the battle between obstetricians and midwives for control of childbirth involves deep-seated views about reproduction and about women. The suspension in 1985 of London obstetrician Wendy Savage for alleged incompetence, carried out on the initiative of her male colleagues, led to a legal inquiry in which these issues were aired in their twentieth-century guise. As Wendy Savage herself said, there is no other explanation for some of what happened other than the term *witch hunt*.

Midwives: The Preferred Sex?

When the fourteenth-century French healer Jacobe Felicie was summoned to a Paris court on a charge of illegal practice, one of her defenses was the need for women to treat women. The first translations of gynecological treatises from the Latin were made so that one woman could "help another in her sykness."

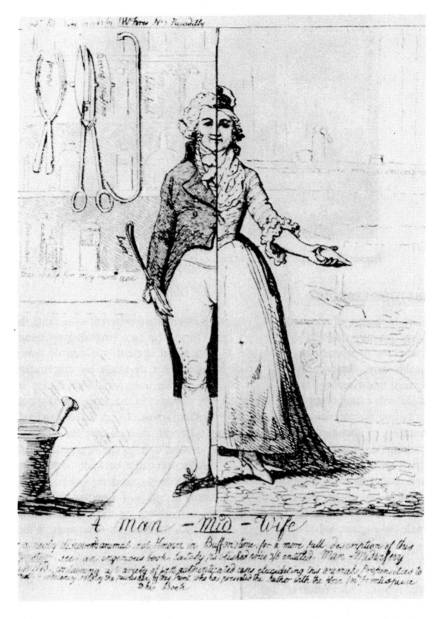

Figure 14 A male midwife. (From S. W. Fores, *Man-midwifery dissected*, London, 1793.)

An identical defense was used to fight the closure of a women's hospital in south London in 1985. History thus provides an argument for the healing arts being more female than male, and it also tells us that it has been the rule and not the exception that women in childbirth have been attended by their own sex.

The twentieth-century introduction of men into nursing and midwifery may thus, not surprisingly, present problems of "patient acceptance." One study in London in 1984, conducted by D. Newbold, found that, while many mothers did not object to male nurses or midwives carrying out procedures such as taking temperatures and measuring blood pressure, more intimate activities, such as inspecting the vulval area, were frequently not regarded as proper tasks for men. In most places, male midwives, like male doctors, have to be chaperoned for intimate examinations.

History gives us messages that we may choose to ignore or reverse; we make history as well as being subject to it. The destiny of midwives in the transition to the twenty-first century remains to be decided. The argument is proceeding on multiple levels all the time. Are pregnancy and childbirth normal or pathological experiences? Who is most at risk when a child is born? Who defines risk anyway? How important are women's own desires about how they give birth, and who should help them to do so?

Between the two models of midwife-managed and doctor-controlled childbirth stands the mother, who wishes to do the best thing for her child and for herself. The problem is that today some people tell her it is impossible for her to do both. Surely a healthy child and a good experience are not the same thing—or are they?

Chapter Three

What Do Midwives Do?

There was no legislation controlling the midwife's work until the nineteenth century. Some countries were even later than this in controlling the sphere of midwifery practice. Legislation was passed in Australia, Norway, and Sweden in 1801; in France in 1803; in Belgium in 1818; in the Federal Republic of Germany, the Netherlands, and the U.S.S.R. in 1865; and in England and Wales in 1902. The shape these national laws took reflected existing differences between countries in what midwives were allowed to do.

Midwifery practice is not only laid down in laws made by national authorities; it is also subject to local institutional regulations. If the midwife works in an institution, she must conform to its rules. These rules are, in most cases, formulated by consultant obstetricians. Usually, midwives have very little say about what goes into them.

Aside from the question of the laws and local regulations governing midwifery work, there is the fundamental issue of the midwife's education and training. What does a person need to be and do to enter a training program as a midwife? What is the content of these programs? Do opportunities exist for further training or for other forms of career extension, such as engagement in research?

All these questions need to be addressed in charting the content of mid-wives' work in different countries today. First, however, we shall take a brief look at some encounters between women and midwives in the real world. The two short accounts that follow come from a Danish antenatal clinic in the mid-1980s.

The midwife is standing up, wearing a white coat over her very smart clothes; she asks the women to sit down. While the midwife is testing the woman's urine, taking her blood pressure, and weighing her, she talks about her own children—twins, born prematurely. The mother doesn't say anything. Then the midwife asks her to lie down on the bed, and she uses ultrasound to find the heartbeat. "I think it's a breech. Do you mind if I examine you internally?" She examines her. "No, it's a head." *Mother:* "I had problems with breastfeeding the first time, but I managed." *Midwife:* "That's fine, then you know you can do it." The woman gets up, gets dressed, says goodbye to the midwife, shakes hands with her, and leaves. This visit takes twelve minutes.

The midwife gets up from her desk, shakes hands with the woman, and asks her to sit down next to the desk. The midwife, still standing up, asks for the mother's specimen of urine so she can test it. The mother starts to talk about her wishes for the delivery: "I don't want the baby to have any eyedrops or any vitamin K injection, please, and I'd like to be in the pool during the first stage. I also want to deliver in the pool." (She is reading from a list she has brought with her.) *Midwife:* "That's not the idea of the pool: to deliver in it. But the other things, there's no problem there. Let's just see what happens, shall we?" The woman is weighed and is now on the bed; the midwife examines her. *Midwife:* "The baby's head is movable, you must call an ambulance if the bag of waters breaks." The woman gets down and says goodbye.

This woman was a nurse, and the midwife seemed irritated by her requests. She tells the researcher afterwards, "It's tiring to get these questions, as if we're not already doing all the right things!" The visit took twenty-five minutes.

LEGISLATION

The bibliographical literature on midwifery legislation in poor, compared even to nursing. This means that ad hoc surveys need to be done to establish the midwife's position in different countries. The World Health Organization (WHO) made one such survey in 1981, covering twenty-four European countries. Appendix 1 looks at the overall coverage by WHO of midwifery in its publications between 1956 and 1983.

The main aim of European legislation on midwifery practice is to define what is meant by the term. The purpose appears to be twofold: first, to limit the scope of the midwife's activities by preventing her from performing duties considered to belong to the medical profession; and, second, to protect the midwife herself from the practice of unqualified people. A great deal of midwifery legislation is, in fact, concerned with what midwives should *not* do.

Midwifery legislation, as we saw in Chapter 1, concentrates on the idea of the midwife as the person qualified to attend normal pregnancies and deliveries. Much greater clarity and detail than this is needed, so that practically all the legal texts contain a list of additional provisions intended to specify what the functions and duties of midwives should and should not be. The legislation varies immensely; for example, in some countries, midwives are allowed to do breech deliveries, in others not. In Belgium, midwives may supervise breech deliveries only in women who have previously had at least one uncomplicated delivery; in Luxembourg, they may do so only when the physician is absent. In most countries, midwives are allowed to perform episiotomies, but in only a few are they permitted to sew them up. Sweden is the only country where midwives are allowed to do vacuum extractions. In Turkey, midwives are not allowed to prescribe any drugs, but must rely on doctors' prescriptions. In the United Kingdom, the rules of the U.K. Central Council for Nursing, Midwifery and Health Visiting (formerly the Central Midwives' Board) list a limited range of drugs that certified midwives are allowed to prescribe.

Several countries have detailed legislation concerning the contents of a midwife's kit, which may in itself prevent her from performing a delivery without a physician. For example, in some countries, midwives are not allowed to include sewing material in the equipment they take to a birth, so, although they are permitted to perform an episiotomy, they cannot repair it. In some countries, legislation covers the midwife's obligation to attend any birth she is asked to handle. In Denmark, for example, a midwife can turn down a request from a woman to attend her birth only "if the midwife is drunk or insane." In the few areas of that country where no midwives are available for home births, a woman can in theory find the closest midwife in the telephone book when she is in labor, and the midwife she calls is then obliged to help her. In the United Kingdom, a midwife also may not refuse, but if she delivers a woman without cover by a local general practitioner, she may be accused of negligence.

The establishment of the European Economic Community (EEC), with its goal of free movement of labor power, has focused attention on these variations. In order for standard directives to apply, differences between the nine EEC member states relating to the sphere of midwifery practice, the status of midwives, entry criteria, length of training, and so on, need to be ironed out. For instance, although the Council of Europe has recommended that there should be no minimum age for entry to a midwifery school, many countries do, in fact, at the moment provide legal minima; these range from sixteen years to twenty-two years. At the other end of the scale, maximum ages are also often laid down, ranging from twenty-seven to fifty years.

Legislation in some countries prohibits men from being midwives, but in Belgium, Denmark, Luxembourg, the Netherlands, and the United Kingdom, men are allowed to enter midwifery. A further important rationale for midwifery legislation is to control entry to, and content of, training programs. Table 4 combines legislative pronouncements on midwifery practice and education for a number of European countries.

Again, the variation, even confusion, is obvious. According to the 1981 WHO survey, *Legislation Concerning Nursing/Midwifery Services and Education:*

> The present legislative situation in Europe can be summarized as follows: the midwifery practice definitions and midwife functions specify, sometimes in great detail, what the midwife's activities comprise and what types of acts are forbidden. A number of regulations specify the different situations where she is obliged to call in a doctor or the activities she is permitted to carry out in case of emergency. The legislative picture in this connection is very different from country to country, and there might have been important reasons which induced the law-maker to formulate elaborate and detailed texts which specify what the midwife is entitled to do and what is forbidden to her.

So far as midwifery training legislation is concerned, this "is notable for the diversity of the current legislative provisions which have been promulgated in order to qualify in this profession." One reason is the ambiguous status of midwifery in relation to nursing: the growing trend for midwifery *not* to be an autonomous profession has meant increasing links with nursing education in many countries.

EDUCATION AND TRAINING

Within Europe today, three types of education and training lead to the qualification of midwife. In direct-entry programs, midwives are trained separately from nurses. The second type are programs in which a nursing diploma is needed before midwifery training can begin. Third, combinations of the first two also exist, in which the first part of the course is spent in nursing studies and the last part studying midwifery. The 1981 WHO survey found seven countries in which there was no route to becoming a midwife other than first training as a nurse: Ireland, Luxembourg, Malta, Norway, Portugal, Spain, and Sweden.

The duration of training ranges from four years (direct entry) in Czechoslovakia and Greece to a one-year postgraduate course for nurses in Ireland, Malta, Norway, Portugal, and Spain. The midwife who wants to qualify further has few possibilities if she is a direct-entry midwife. Only a few countries have postbasic midwifery training for direct-entry midwives. A nurse-midwife has whatever opportunities exist locally in nursing.

To give a slightly more detailed picture of what goes on under the heading

Table 4 **Practical Experience Required for Qualification as a Midwife in Selected European Countries, 1981**

Country	The midwifery student:
Austria	must provide "midwifery assistance" at 30 deliveries
Belgium	must have "personally carried out" 100 prenatal examinations and 40 deliveries
Ireland	must have "personally conducted" at least 30 deliveries and have obtained experience of at least 70 antenatal examinations
Luxembourg	must "perform" at least 30 normal deliveries and at least 100 prenatal and postnatal examinations, and "provide assistance" at 30 dystocic deliveries
Norway	must "attend and assist" at a minimum of 50 deliveries

Source: WHO, 1981.

of midwifery training, we describe what happens in one country: the Netherlands.

There are three midwifery training schools in the Netherlands, each accepting (in the early 1980s) about twenty students a year. Each school is run by an obstetrician and a midwife; 93 percent of student midwives are direct entrants, the other 7 percent being nurses or occasionally medical students. Students have to be at least nineteen years of age and are rarely accepted if over thirty-five years of age. Training lasts three years for all entrants. About a third of the training period is spent in the antenatal area, somewhat less than a third on the labor ward, and only 4 percent of the time doing community midwifery. Students learn not only basic subjects, such as anatomy and physiology, but also ethics, family planning, sociology, and social medicine. About one in four students drops out; this is said to be because of the high standards they are required to meet.

PRACTICE

In another WHO survey carried out for the 1985 report, *Having a Baby in Europe,* questionnaires were completed by twenty-three European countries describing official services for pregnancy and birth. The resulting information gives some insight into what midwives actually do, as opposed to what they are legally permitted to do.

The general rule appears to be that midwives do less than they are allowed. Eighteen countries said they had regulations concerning who provides preventive care during pregnancy. In twenty-two countries, midwives were legally permitted to participate in pregnancy care, but only in nineteen did they actually do so. Almost all countries described a responsibility for care during pregnancy that is shared between midwives and physicians. According to the report:

> Most questionnaire respondents admitted that it is not known precisely what the midwives actually do. Many respondents volunteered the information that the role of midwives in care during pregnancy (and birth) is changing and that their profession is, in fact, threatened for a number of reasons, including the increasing role of physicians, especially obstetricians, in the routine care of uncomplicated cases; the replacement of midwives by nurses; and the moving of midwives into hospitals. . . . There is a trend towards enlarging the role of physicians in preventive care during pregnancy, although only four countries reported that physicians are solely responsible for pregnancy care.

In some cases, who should give care how many times is exactly defined; in one country, ten visits to the midwife and two visits to the doctor are specified; in another, twenty visits to the midwife and ten to the doctor.

In a few countries midwives go to pregnant women's homes, but this happens mostly when the woman does not turn up in the antenatal clinic. In eastern European countries, much home visiting during pregnancy is done. In these cases, however, it is done not by midwives but by health visitors. Most countries have one group of midwives working in antenatal care, a different group providing birth services, and yet another group giving postnatal care. In only a few countries—e.g., Denmark and the Netherlands—does the midwife work both in the health center or home and in the hospital. In the Federal Republic of Germany, in Italy, and to some degree in Greece, Morocco, and Norway, midwives are relatively uninvolved in antenatal care. Antenatal care is given by midwives in Denmark, France, the Netherlands, Sweden, and the United Kingdom, but doctors are also involved. In southern European countries, antenatal care has been totally taken over by doctors. In the U.S.S.R., doctors and midwives work together. The midwife takes the blood pressure, does the different tests, and then she is there when the doctor examines the woman. She is more of an assistant; it's the doctor's decision that counts in the end—although, if the midwife says something or has a suggestion to make, it will be considered.

In Norway, midwives are fighting to be allowed into antenatal care, which is dominated by general practitioners. In Sweden, however, midwives work quite independently in antenatal clinics. They even carry out ultrasound scanning themselves.

While many countries have official guidelines for care during pregnancy, most of these have to do with the structure rather than the content of care. If the guidelines describe what happens during antenatal examinations, they give no information on the extent to which the care actually given in practice coincides with the care thus prescribed. Some countries do mention that midwives have advantages as providers of pregnancy care, since they are "sensitive to social needs and to providing health promotion."

So far as birth is concerned, the 1985 WHO survey found that, in seventeen of twenty-one countries providing this information, the midwife is the birth attendant in uncomplicated births. In ten of these seventeen countries, midwives attend 100 percent of the births. In only six countries are physicians said to be present at most uncomplicated births. In only one country (the Netherlands) do midwives give total continuity of care for women having babies, and this is only for 40 percent of the women; in the rest of the countries, continuity of care does not exist.

It is difficult, if not impossible, to account for these international differences in midwifery care. One factor, however, undoubtedly has to do with the type of health care system and its financing. The basic distinction is between a *monopolistic* health care system, with one publicly provided source of health care, and a *pluralist* system, with more than one source of care and usually including some privately provided care. Midwives seem to retain their autonomy over uncomplicated births in countries with monopolistic health care systems. In the others, although the midwife may be entitled by law to deliver uncomplicated births, there are various incentives, some of them financial, for physicians to take over.

INDEPENDENT PRACTITIONERS?

Clearly, the idea of the midwife as an independent practitioner has been considerably modified by law, custom, and interprofessional politics in many countries today. The range is wide: from absolutely no autonomy in many eastern European countries to semi-independent practitioners in the Netherlands and some Scandinavian countries. Differences in autonomy can also be seen within a country; for example, midwives generally have more autonomy in small hospitals than in large ones. If we look at the extent to which midwives participate in decision making, the differences are not so large; there are few midwives at this level anywhere.

One consequence of the new interest in the status and role of the midwife has been more research into the content of midwives' work, and particularly the limits of different work settings, which affect the capacity to behave as independent practitioners. One such study, by an English midwife-researcher, Rosemary Methven (1982), took one standard item in antenatal care—the booking history—and examined the extent to which midwives' performance in taking this was shaped by predetermined conditions, including the format of the case notes. Methven found that midwives asked about the issue said case notes were important. This led midwives to ignore other areas of crucial significance to midwifery care:

For instance, in every interview the date of any previous confinements was required. However, midwives in the study did not enquire as to the present age of any children or whether the mother was also caring for children by a different marriage . . . children who had been adopted or were currently being fostered. Thus, no picture of the mother's current workload during pregnancy emerged. . . .

Midwives did enquire about the type of delivery a mother had had previously, but they did not always enquire as to the reason for that delivery, and seldom asked about such details as episiotomy and stitches or how a perineal or abdominal wound may have healed. Similarly, where it was required on the notes, midwives asked the mother how she intended to feed her next baby, but did not question her about any previous experience of feeding. . . .

Questions relating to a mother's emotional or psychological response to pregnancy and childbirth did not feature during the interviews observed.

Methven concluded from these findings that the antenatal booking interview as currently conducted is obstetric rather than midwifery in its orientation. It fits a medical rather than a nursing-midwifery model of care. This means that midwives are "unintentionally regarding the mother as an obstetric object rather than a person with hopes and fears, views and opinions, personality and relationships within a unique social context."

Here, to illustrate what Methven is talking about, is one booking interview recorded by Ann Oakley in 1974 in a London antenatal clinic:

Midwife: You're Mrs. Morgan, and you're twenty-six years old, you were born on 21 July 1948, and you're (*reading referral letter from doctor*) RC—what does that mean?

Mother: I should imagine it's Roman Catholic, but I'm not a Catholic; my husband is.

Midwife: Your husband is David Morgan, and he lives at the same address?

Mother: I hope so!

Midwife: Your doctor's name is Dr. Kahn, and his telephone number is . . .

Mother: I don't know his telephone number.

Midwife: And you were married in 1972, and your maiden name was Cunningham; you're British?

Mother: Yes.

Midwife: Are you still at work?

Mother: Yes.

Midwife: What do you do?

Mother: I'm a florist.

Midwife: Your husband's occupation?

Mother: He's a banqueting porter—shall I spell that for you?

Midwife: Yes, please! Your father's occupation?

Mother: He's dead, but he was a market gardener.

Midwife: And you've never been divorced, widowed, or separated?

Mother: No.

Midwife: And your last menstrual period was the sixteenth of August?
Mother: Yes.
Midwife: And it was an ordinary period, it wasn't shorter than usual? The same amount of bleeding?
Mother: Yes.
Midwife: How long do you usually bleed for?
Mother: I'd only just come off the pill.
Midwife: Oh, I see!
Mother: I came off the pill in June.
Midwife: And when did you go on the pill?
Mother: In March 1972.
Midwife: And did you come off specifically to have a baby?
Mother: Yes.
Midwife: You were lucky, weren't you? You didn't have to wait long! And were your periods regular?
Mother: Yes.
Midwife: How long did they last?
Mother: Four to five days usually, when I was off the pill.
Midwife: How long did you have between?
Mother: Twenty-six or twenty-seven days, usually.
Midwife: Now I want to ask a few questions about your past obstetric history.
Mother: I haven't got one!
Midwife: Is this your first pregnancy?
Mother: Yes.
Midwife: You've never had a miscarriage or a termination?
Mother: No.
Midwife: Right. Your past medical history now.
Mother: I haven't got one of those either!
Midwife: Oh. Have you ever had german measles?
Mother: No, I haven't had anything.
Midwife: Scarlet fever, chicken pox?
Mother: No.
Midwife: How did you escape? Heart disorders? Chest disorders? Have you been in contact with tuberculosis at any time?
Mother: Not so far as I know.
Midwife: Do you suffer from asthma or bronchitis?
Mother: No.
Midwife: You've never had cystitis—urinary tract infection?
Mother: I had a slight infection a year ago, which they diagnosed as thrush.
Midwife: Gosh, you're remarkably healthy! Have you ever had cortisone or steroid pills?
Mother: No.
Midwife: Are you taking anything at the moment?
Mother: Only what the doctor gave me.
Midwife: Are you allergic to any drugs—for instance, penicillin?

Mother: No.

Midwife: Are you allergic to Elastoplast?[1]

Mother: No.

Midwife: Have you had any operations—appendix, D and C?[2]

Mother: No.

Midwife: Have you had any accidents?

Mother: Not serious ones.

Midwife: To your pelvis? Fractures?

Mother: No.

Midwife: To your chest?

Mother: Well, what sort of accidents? I've had minor accidents—a cut finger, that sort of thing. Interesting, aren't I?

Midwife: Have you ever had any x rays, of your kidneys, for instance?

Mother: No.

Midwife: Have you ever been to an infertility clinic?

Mother: No, I didn't have a chance!

Midwife: Are you anemic?

Mother: No.

Midwife: Is there any history of diabetes in your family?

Mother: Only my grandmother.

Midwife: Was that when she was old?

Mother: Yes, right at the end, before she died.

Midwife: Any twins in the family?

Mother: My cousin's wife.

Midwife: That's not close enough—they have to be related. No one in your husband's family has had twins, tuberculosis, epilepsy?

Mother: No to all those questions! No, the only thing they've got is asthma.

Midwife: How do you feel at the moment? Are you tired at all?

Mother: Yes, by the evening.

Midwife: Are you eating well?

Mother: Yes, too well; I got told off the other day!

Midwife: By your doctor, you mean?

Mother: Yes *(laughs)*.

Midwife: Are you sleeping well?

Mother: Yes.

Midwife: Have you had any blood loss from the vagina?

Mother: No.

Midwife: Bowels all right?

Mother: I get constipation, but it usually sorts itself out.

Midwife: Nausea?

Mother: Yes.

Midwife: When?

Mother: At the beginning, before I ever went to the doctor. He gave me pills, and I've just come off them and I'm all right.

---

[1] Elastoplast® is a type of dressing.

[2] D and C stands for "dilatation and curettage."

Midwife: So you think your general condition is healthy?

Mother: Yes.

Midwife: Have you been to the dentist?

Mother: Yes, I finished the last lot of treatment a few weeks ago.

Midwife: You know that dental treatment's free during pregnancy, don't you?[3] I would take the opportunity of going again if I were you.

Mother: I will.

Midwife: It's important, too, in pregnancy, because if you get any infections, they tend to spread. Have you had a chest x ray recently?

Mother: No, never.

Midwife: Cervical smear?

Mother: Before, when I'd been on the pill about fifteen months, about the end of last year, I think it was.

Midwife: None of the babies born in your family have had anything wrong with them—six toes, six fingers, that sort of thing?

Mother: One of my husband's sisters is very backward, that's all, but that's only one of ten, that's not bad, is it?

Midwife: Is she very backward?

Mother: No, she's a bit slow, always has been.

Midwife: Is she out at work?

Mother: Yes, she works in a hospital, as a—what do you call them?

Midwife: Nursing auxiliary?

Mother: That's right.

Midwife: Ah, that's all right. Do you know at all if you'd like to breastfeed or bottle feed?

Mother: I'd like to breastfeed if I possibly can, at least at the beginning. It's nicer if you can, I think.

Midwife: Yes, after all, it's natural, and it's better for the baby. We ask you now, because you can start to prepare yourself to breastfeed from the middle of your pregnancy. The doctor will examine your nipples. Have you been depressed at all during the pregnancy?

Mother: A bit.

Midwife: Seriously depressed?

Mother: No, not really. At the beginning a bit, because there's nothing to show for it.

Midwife: Well, I've never met anyone as healthy.

In this encounter between a midwife and a first-time mother, the questions probing the mother's medical history seem endless, and the amount of social and personal information collected is very small in comparison. In her study, Methven found that the way in which booking histories are taken rarely makes it possible for a mother and midwife to establish a relationship—although midwives more often than mothers believe that they have, in fact, accomplished this. Perhaps there is a need to idealize the real world of midwifery practice.

[3]Under the British National Health Service.

Two large studies of the midwife's role have been conducted in the United Kingdom: a 1983 study on the role and responsibilities of the midwife, by Sarah Robinson and her colleagues at the Department of Health, Nursing Research Unit, Chelsea College, London, and a 1985 study on policy and practice in midwifery by Jo Garcia and colleagues from the National Perinatal Epidemiology Unit in Oxford. Both were national studies, sampling the views and experiences of midwives and other health professionals all over the country. They covered many aspects of midwifery and so are too extensive for us to do them justice here, but it is important to refer to some of their main findings. These provide the much-coveted hard data to back up more isolated and intimate accounts of the midwife's work.

The Nursing Research Unit study came to three main conclusions about the work of midwives.

1 A substantial proportion of midwives practiced in situations in which they were not required to exercise fully the degree of clinical responsibility for which the midwife is trained (this was particularly the case for antenatal care).

2 Medical staff were significantly less likely than midwives to indicate that midwives made decisions concerning normal antepartum and intrapartum care.

3 The proportion of midwives who did fully exercise clinical responsibility differed significantly by the type of practice situation in which they worked.

Tables 5–10 flesh out these statements. Table 5 shows responsibility for a standard antenatal procedure—abdominal examination—that lies well within the ordinary clinical skills of all midwives. The most common practice in consultant obstetric units, however, is that the midwife examines the mother, and this examination is then repeated by a doctor. Only 4 percent of the respondents said

Table 5 Hospital Midwives Working in Consultant Obstetric Units: Responsibility for Abdominal Examination

Responsibility for abdominal examination	Percentage[a] of respondents (N = 634)
Usually carried out by midwife only	4
Usually carried out by doctor only	33
Carried out by midwife but usually repeated by a doctor	57
No answer	5
Total	100

[a]Rounded off.

Source: Robinson et al., 1983. Copyright © 1983 by Department of Health and Social Security, United Kingdom.

Table 6   Community Midwives: Responsibility for Abdominal Examination

Responsibility for abdominal examination	Percentage of respondents (*N* = 1159)
Usually carried out by midwife only	14
Usually carried out by doctor only	17
Carried out by midwife but usually repeated by a doctor	49
Other/variable	15
No answer	5
Total	100

Source: Robinson et al., 1983. Copyright © 1983 by Department of Health and Social Security, United Kingdom.

Table 7   Hospital Midwives: Responsibility for Management of Normal Labor by Type of Unit

Management of normal labor	Percentage of all respondents (*N* = 2136)	Percentage[a] of respondents working in:		
		Consultant units	Integrated general practitioner units	Separate general practitioner units
Patients in normal labor are cared for by a midwife and not examined by a doctor unless the midwife requests it	82	80	83	95
All patients are examined by a doctor on admission and then normal labor is managed by midwives unless problems arise	11	12	11	3
All patients are examined by a doctor on admission, visited regularly through labor, and decisions as to management are made by a doctor	4	5	2	1
No answer	3	4	3	1
Total	100	100	100	100

[a]Rounded off.
Source: Robinson et al., 1983. Copyright © 1983 by Department of Health and Social Security, United Kingdom.

Table 8   Hospital Midwives: Decision Making on When to Carry out Vaginal Examinations

When to do vaginal examinations in normal labor	Percentage of all respondents (N = 1984)	Percentage[a] of respondents working in:		
		Consultant units	Integrated general practitioner units	Separate general practitioner units
Decision usually made by midwife	56	47	73	93
Decision usually made by a doctor	1	1	–	–
There is a unit policy that specifies procedure	41	49	24	5
No answer	3	3	4	1
Total	100	100	100	100

[a]Rounded off.
Source: Robinson et al., 1983. Copyright © 1983 by Department of Health and Social Security, United Kingdom.

that the midwife normally carried responsibility for this examination on her own.

Table 6 shows the same procedure in the somewhat different setting of antenatal clinics in the community. Here, by contrast, midwives are much more likely to behave autonomously, and 14 percent said that abdominal examina-

Table 9   Hospital Midwives: Views on Their Ability to Give Support to Women in Labor, by Type of Unit

Able to give support to women in labor that the midwife feels is necessary	Percentage of all respondents (N = 2136)	Percentage[a] of respondents working in:		
		Consultant units	Integrated general practitioner units	Separate general practitioner units
Yes	71	68	76	94
No	28	30	22	4
No answer	2	2	2	2
Total	100	100	100	100

[a]Rounded off.
Source: Robinson et al., 1983. Copyright © 1983 by Department of Health and Social Security, United Kingdom.

Table 10   Hospital Medical Staff and Midwives Working in Consultant Units:
Percentage of Respondents Who Said Decisions Were Made by the Midwife

Decision	Percentage of respondents who said decisions were usually made by the midwife	
	Hospital medical staff	Midwives in consultant units
When to carry out examination in normal labor	33	47
At what point during labor to rupture membranes	30	56
Whether to give intramuscular analgesics in normal labor	66	79
Whether to use continuous monitoring machine in normal labor	12	37
Whether to do episiotomy	72	94

Source: Robinson et al., 1983. Copyright © 1983 by Department of Health and Social Security, United Kingdom.

tions are normally carried out by midwives on their own. This is clear evidence that the midwife's autonomy is affected by clinical setting. Further support for this appears in Table 7, which looks at the management of normal labor in consultant obstetric units and in two types of general practitioner unit: those that are integrated with and those that are separate from the hospital. Here, 82% of the sample as a whole agreed that it is normal practice in their places of work for women in normal labor to be cared for by midwives, with doctor consultation only if the midwife thinks it necessary. This model of care, which preserves the principle of midwife autonomy, is most likely to operate in the separate general practitioner units and least likely to be found in consultant obstetric units. In fact, one in twenty midwives working in consultant units described the usual procedure as a doctor seeing all women on admission, regular monitoring by a doctor throughout labor, and all management decisions also being a medical prerogative. Table 8 echoes this for one particular decision: carrying out vaginal examinations during labor. Less than 50 percent of consultant unit midwives said it was up to them to decide when this should be done, compared to more than 90 percent of those working in separate general practitioner units.

Other work confirms the picture of the presence of senior medical and nursing staff inhibiting the practice of midwifery as an independent profession. In a small study in northern England, midwife Mavis Kirkham observed labors and interviewed mothers and midwives about the role of the midwife in child-birth care. She found that the aspect of midwifery most often stressed as valuable by mothers was that the midwife should be someone "who gave them information with which to orientate themselves in their labour." In line with this, most midwives also emphasized that giving information was a crucial part of their job. An important inhibiting factor, however, was the senior staff: "I repeatedly saw," says Kirkham, "student midwives explaining the results of a vaginal examination to the patient immediately after a sister or nursing officer had left the room. Likewise the sister would explain after the doctor had left the room." Sometimes the explanation would consist of a detailed account of a particular procedure, but sometimes it was a matter of explaining why a procedure was done, which in turn often meant describing the policy of that unit or consultant.

Table 9 displays some statistics related to a theme that recurs constantly in any modern description of midwifery work: the extent to which midwives feel able to give the necessary personal support to women in labor. Less than three quarters of the respondents in the Nursing Research Unit study felt able to do this, but the percentage was considerably higher in the separate general practitioner unit setting than in the consultant obstetric units.

Finally, from the Nursing Research Unit study, we have Table 10, which shows some interesting discrepancies between what doctors and midwives respectively regard as legitimate midwifery work. For the five procedures listed in the table, considerably more midwives than doctors think that decisions are made by midwives. Midwives see themselves as independent practitioners to a far greater extent than doctors are prepared to allow.

The second national study of midwifery in the United Kingdom looked specifically at the thorny—but for midwives extremely important—issue of the relationship between policy and practice. The aim of this study was, first, to establish to what extent consultant units responsible for delivering women have policies dictating the frequency with which certain procedures should be used and who should carry out these procedures. Second, it attempted to see whether such policies, where they did exist, were reflected in actual practice. This issue of the relationship between local institutional policy and actual midwifery practice is a critical one for many midwives today. In the United Kingdom, for example, midwives are often allowed more autonomy by the laws and statutes governing their practice than by their particular institutional setting.. This complicates clinical decision making for midwives, who are held legally responsible for their actions even when their treatment of an individual women is determined by local hospital policy and goes against the midwife's own clinical opinion. In such cases, a midwife may be called on to defend a decision that was not hers in the first place.

Figures 15–19 pick out some of the results of the Oxford study of policy and practice in midwifery. First is a subject explored in the Nursing Research Unit study: vaginal examinations in labor. According to the information in Figure 15, 30 percent of consultant units have no policy on this, while 36 percent examine on a fixed and 34 percent on a flexible schedule. Midwives

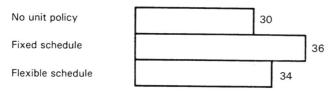

No unit policy 30

Fixed schedule 36

Flexible schedule 34

Figure 15 Percentage of consultant units (*N* = 217) and their policy on frequency of vaginal examination in labor. (From Garcia et al., 1985.)

working in units where there is a policy thus need to be aware of it and adjust their behavior accordingly.

Figures 16 and 17 relate to the uncomfortable question of pubic shaves; they demonstrate that, whatever the status of the scientific evidence on this, 38 percent of consultant units still have a policy of either complete or partial shaves for women in labor. Figure 17 shows that 41 percent of respondents estimated that from more than half to almost all women continue to be shaved.

Figures 18 and 19 describe the use of electronic fetal monitoring (EFM) in labor. Twenty-eight percent of units have a policy of monitoring every woman, either throughout labor or for part of it. Forty-nine percent claim to monitor high risk cases only. Eleven percent say that "consultants vary," which, given the current debate about the value of monitoring, does not seem surprising. Yet these policies, translated into practice, mean that 32 percent of units say "almost all" women are monitored, and a further 38 percent reckon that "more than half" are. This team of researchers concludes by saying that "an individual midwife will have to consider many factors when making decisions about her practice. She must be aware of policies, guidelines, procedures, standing orders from consultants, the statutory Midwives Rules and the Midwife's Code

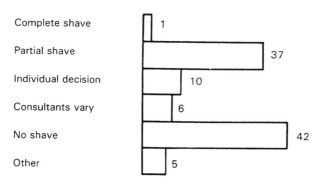

Complete shave 1

Partial shave 37

Individual decision 10

Consultants vary 6

No shave 42

Other 5

Figure 16 Percentage of consultant units (*N* = 220) with shaving policies on admissions in labor. (From Garcia et al., 1985.)

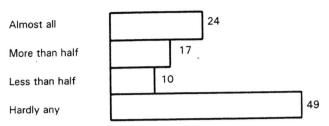

Figure 17   Percentage of consultant units (*N* = 208) and proportion of women having some sort of shave. (From Garcia et al., 1985.)

of Practice. She will be aware of pressure from women to have some control in childbearing at the same time as she seeks to provide safe and effective care."

An impossible dilemma? As a number of facts conspire to reduce the midwife's autonomy, many midwives feel they are not capable of giving independent care. Further decline in the midwife's role is then a self-fulfilling prophecy. There are, however, various ways around this problem. One example is the organizational "innovation" of midwife-only clinics. These are clinics staffed only by midwives, who either see women who have been screened by doctors and determined to be at low risk or do this screening themselves, referring women to doctors where necessary. In the United Kingdom, according to one midwife working in a midwife-only clinic, "as our midwives' clinic progresses, so the confidence of the midwives who run it grows. Seeing the same woman month by month and then week by week shows the midwife that she is perfectly capable of giving antenatal care, and this makes her more alert to signs that all is not going well, because she knows the woman so well. Her confidence is increased by the attitude of the women she sees; they respect and trust her and look forward to seeing her."

ARE MIDWIVES SAFE?

Ever since physicians and midwives began fighting for the control of childbirth, recurrent questions have been asked. Is it safe to leave most pregnancies and childbirths to the care of midwives? What effect does midwifery care have on perinatal and maternal mortality and morbidity? How, if at all, does it affect rates of intervention? How does midwifery care compare with doctor care, not only in terms of effectiveness but according to the important measure of satisfaction of the women who are cared for?

In 1985, the U.S. Office of Technology Assessment carried out a technology assessment of nursing and midwifery care. Some possible outcomes of this care are naturally very difficult to assess. For example, there are as yet no standard measures of the general health-promoting effects of midwife (or any other) care. Nevertheless, the report concluded that "evidence is abundant that

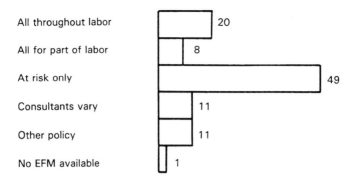

Figure 18 Percentage of consultant units (N = 218) with policy for electronic fetal monitoring (EFM) in labor. (From Garcia et al., 1985.)

certified nurse-midwives manage normal pregnancies safely as well as, if not better than, physicians." Midwife care is associated with less medication in labor and delivery and shorter hospital stays for labor and delivery. The report found that health care provided by nurses or midwives was characterized by better communication and counseling skills than those provided by doctors. A study by H. B. Perry in 1980 showed that 88 percent of women were very satisfied with their midwives, whereas only 45 percent claimed this level of satisfaction with their obstetricians. Of women delivered by midwives, none subsequently said they would have preferred to have had a doctor for delivery. Some of the women whose babies were delivered by doctors felt afterward that they would have preferred midwife care.

One problem with, comparing the safety and effectiveness of midwife care with those of doctor care is that midwives and doctors tend to care for different groups of women who have different levels of risk in childbirth. What is needed is a study using random assignment, so that women are allocated randomly either to physician or to midwife care. The results of these two forms of care could then be compared in the knowledge that the two groups of clients are

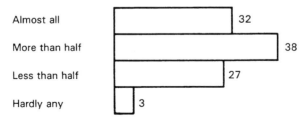

Figure 19 Percentage of consultant units (N = 208) with estimated proportion of electronic fetal monitoring (EFM) in labor. (From Garcia et al., 1985.)

likely to be the same. There are a few studies of this kind. In the earliest of these, Lillian Runnerstrom compared the care given by nurse-midwives with that provided by obstetric residents to a population of 1773 women. No differences in mortality or obvious morbidities were found. Runnerstrom did find that nurse-midwives gave analgesic drugs to more of the women in their care than did doctors, but they gave smaller doses. Their clients had shorter labors and a lower chance of undergoing an episiotomy. Ninety percent of them had a normal spontaneous delivery, compared with 42 percent among physician-delivered women. The second study, by Slome et al. in 1976, had similar findings; 83 percent of women looked after by nurse-midwives had a normal spontaneous delivery, as against 62 percent of women cared for by obstetric staff.

A somewhat different study was reported by David Olds et al. in 1986. This was an intervention study, in which the intervention consisted of using nurse-midwives to make home visits to a socially disadvantaged population (selected on a random basis and thus compared with an equivalent control group). Olds found that nurse-midwives seemed to be particularly effective in improving the outcome of pregnancy (using birth weight as a measure of this) for pregnant adolescents and for the babies of women who smoked. A French study, by Nadine Spira et al., also examined the effects of home visiting, this time as a way of providing normal antenatal midwifery care. The result of this scheme was a significant improvement for women with "social" risks only, but results were not so good for those with clear medical risks.

Few studies look at both effectiveness and how women feel about the service they get. One that did combine these measures was the study by Reid et al. in Glasgow comparing the delivery of antenatal care in the community with that of a centralized hospital clinic. All clinical outcomes of pregnancy were essentially the same in the two groups. The rate of low birth weight babies was somewhat smaller in the women cared for in the community (8 percent as opposed to 13 percent). The women who attended the community clinic received more midwife-centered care and continuity of care. This continuity was an important element in the higher satisfaction women reported with the community service.

The "know-your-midwife" scheme pioneered by Caroline Flint in England is an attempt to provide this feature, which is so often mentioned by women as important: the opportunity to form a relationship with one or a small number of care providers instead of being passed from one anonymous face and pair of hands to another. Flint set up her scheme in a hospital in south London as a randomized controlled trial of continuity of care, which would be able to examine whether continuity of care could in itself have an effect on clinical outcomes of pregnancy as well as allowing mothers to feel happier about the care they received. For a period of about two years, a team of four midwives gave nearly all antenatal, intrapartum, and postpartum care to 250 women a year. When the data were analyzed at the end of this time, the "know-your-midwife" group had fewer antenatal admissions, fewer interventions, less analgesia, less acceleration of labor, and a greater chance of having a normal, spontaneous delivery than the control group, which received standard antenatal care. The experimental group were more satisfied with their antenatal care, felt more prepared for labor and motherhood, and found labor a more positive experience. Table 11 shows the distribution of feelings of control in labor between the two groups in the study; the women in the experimental group were much more likely to report feeling "very much in control."

There are two ways of interpreting these findings. One is in terms of how midwives, as opposed to physicians, relate to the women in their care; midwives can provide a service that is more client-centered and more client-sensitive. This is not, of course, to say that midwifery care is invariably more humane in this sense. Some women's accounts of their childbirth experiences bring out the failure even of continuity of care to guarantee a feeling of "being cared for"; hierarchies within midwifery and aspects of midwifery training can act against the chances of individual midwives being genuinely "*with* women." Midwives have direct power over women giving birth, and sometimes in the exercise of this power they lose sight of their capacity to be sensitive to the woman's experience. Midwives are human beings, and human beings can abuse, as well as use constructively, their power over others.

A second way of interpreting the findings of the "know-your-midwife" scheme is in terms of a social model of childbirth. Childbirth is a biological process that is located in a social setting; mind and body, emotions and biological processes, and body and environment all interact. What the pregnant woman enjoys—whether it be a good meal or sensitive antenatal care—is actually good for her and for her fetus. What midwives provide is clinically effective social support. There is "hard" evidence that social support is not only enjoyed by the women receiving it, but also makes a difference to the outcome of pregnancy. The studies in this field are escalating fast. Table 12 shows some of the most

Table 11 Feelings of Control in Labor: Women in the "Know-Your-Midwife" Scheme Compared with Those in the Control Group

Feelings of control	"Know-your-midwife" group (%)	Control group (%)
Very much in control	42	24
Fairly in control	36	43
Not much/no control	22	33
Total	100	100
	(N = 246)	(N = 225)

Source: Flint & Poulengeris, 1987.

Table 12   Percentage of Women Having Perinatal Problems during Labor, with and without Social Support

	Percentage of women receiving no social support (N = 249)	Percentage of women receiving social support (N = 168)
Caesarean section	17	7
Meconium staining	18	13
Asphyxia	3	2
Oxytocin	13	2
Analgesia	4	1
Forceps	3	1
Other	1	1
No problems	41	73
Total	100	100

Source: Klaus et al., 1986.

impressive results, from one of the simplest studies—an intervention study in Guatemala in which women were randomly assigned either to receive the support of a lay companion in labor (previously unknown to them) or not. The table shows clearly that social support in labor is a good thing. It is equally obvious from much of the material surveyed in this chapter that social support is at the heart of the midwife model of care; it lies behind the idea of being "*with* women," which the settings and conditions of modern obstetric care make it increasingly hard for midwives to provide.

Chapter Four

Childbirth Today

Childbirth in Europe in the 1980s has become a much debated issue—a focus of intense and complex power struggles, a place of great pain for some, a financial gold mine for others. For some women, it remains a yearly event beyond their control; for others, it has the status of a desired and planned event; while yet others may want to become mothers but find biology defeats them. Resources for birth—economic, social, and human—are very unevenly allocated. The kind of care given differs from place to place. Survival rates for both babies and mothers also differ from country to country and do not necessarily reflect the amount spent on professional health services. In short, childbirth is a very complex scene.

Who gives birth in today's Europe? Generally, the more developed a country, the fewer children women have. Some women today choose to have no children at all; they may want to have control over their own lives, undisturbed by the responsibility of parenthood, and they may not want to bring a child into a world marked by such an uncertain future and so much violence and evident unhappiness. Some women delay childbearing so as to make sure of their place in the public world of work. In southern Europe, the situation is different.

There, to have children is still generally considered a gift from God and a help in old age, though in the industrial centers the more "modern" pattern may hold.

Here is a description of an ordinary birth as it happens now in large hospitals in the more developed countries of Europe. The significance of this account relates not only to the present but to the future, for this is the way childbirth is going. It is what will happen in more and more places unless current trends are halted or reversed.

Carla Green is in labor with her first baby. She is having contractions ten minutes apart. She calls the hospital and is instructed to call an ambulance to take her to the hospital. When she and her husband arrive, she is asked to don hospital clothes and is put to bed. Her temperature and pulse are taken, a doctor asks her how she is and examines her, and she is taken to the labor ward. Here, a fetal monitor is attached, and blood tests are taken. Her husband is dressed in special clothes, as he is assumed to be contaminated with bacteria. She is given some pain relief. The pain relief makes her feel sleepy. During her labor, a midwife or a nurse is there some of the time, checking her every fifteen minutes, examining her internally every hour or so. The doctor comes to see her every now and then and gives orders designed to ensure that the labor progresses rapidly.

Carla Green's membranes are ruptured, and an internal scalp electrode is inserted so the baby's heartbeat is easier to follow. Her husband washes her forehead with a cloth. Because by now she's complaining a lot, she's offered an epidural anesthetic, which leaves her without any feeling of what's going on from her waist down. When she's ready to push, she finds it difficult and needs to be helped by the doctor with forceps—but not until she's moved to a second room, effectively an operating theater, and lifted onto another bed with great difficulty, because she finds it very uncomfortable to be moved at that point. Then she's given an episiotomy, and the baby is pulled out. (See Figure 20.) After the mother has held her new daughter briefly, the baby is given to the pediatrician, because she is slow to respond. The father is sent out of the room, because there's only enough space for the twelve other people who are needed in the room at this stage. Several of these are students of medicine and midwifery.

The baby is taken away to the neonatal unit, just in case. The parents are told not to worry. Carla Green is now on her back with her legs in stirrups; she has been like that for quite a while. Half the people in the room are looking in a very interested way at her bottom, while the doctor is explaining to the students how to sew her together again. He says to her, "We'll be careful and make sure we don't sew you totally together, I'm sure Mr. Green wouldn't appreciate that!" (general laughter).

In the meantime, Mr. Green has been urged to accompany the pediatrician to the neonatal unit, so he can reassure his wife that the baby is all right: "We

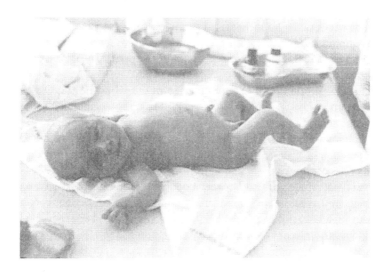

Figure 20 The baby at the hospital.

are all for openness here, we think information is very important in this hospital." On the way to the unit, the pediatrician has a man-to-man talk with the
father about all the new technological advances in this field. "I'm sure your
baby will make it," he says reassuringly. If the pediatrician is a woman, she
may suggest that the father give one finger to the baby to hold: "Notice how
strong your baby is; she immediately knows you're her father. Go and tell your
wife that we're taking good care of the baby; she should concentrate on getting
a good rest."

Back in the delivery room, Carla Green is now "as good as new, maybe
even better" according to the doctor who sewed up her episiotomy. She is lifted
into a clean bed. She still can't feel anything from the waist down, but she does
feel exhausted. She's given a cup of tea and then taken to the postnatal ward,
where her husband meets her before going home.

A few hours later, the baby is declared "okay" and taken to the mother, as
the staff believe in the need "to support early mother/child bonding." However,
the baby is asleep, and the mother is tired and also wants to sleep. The staff
offer to mind the baby while the mother gets some rest. Unfortunately, while
Carla Green is getting her much deserved and wished-for rest, the baby wakes
up and is very hungry. Since the staff want to be considerate and let the mother
sleep, they feed the baby with a bottle. Later, when the mother wakes up and
tries to breastfeed, the baby screams.

On the fifth day, the sutures are removed. Carla Green feels very sore
"down there," but she's told this is quite normal and it will soon disappear. Her
husband comes to take her home. She leaves a nice bottle of wine for the

obstetrician and the ward staff, including the midwife on the delivery ward. In a note to the obstetrician she writes, "Thank you for your excellent treatment."

As a matter of fact, just after the baby was born, Carla Green had grabbed the obstetrician's hand and said, with tears in her eyes, "Thank you so much, I never would have been able to do it without you."

Tables 13–17 and Figure 21 are taken from the World Health Organization (WHO) report, *Having a Baby in Europe*. They show numbers of antenatal visits recommended and made in the various countries that took part in a survey of the contemporary maternity care scene, screening tests carried out in pregnancy, operative births, women's choices during birth, bonding procedures, and maternity leave provisions. The data, which were collected in 1981–82, describe a considerable variation between countries in matters that are supposedly determined by hard scientific evidence—for instance, how commonly women need instrumental assistance at delivery, or the desirable frequency of examinations and specific screening procedures during pregnancy. These data also illustrate the general "medicalization" of childbirth today and the limited extent to which women's own choices about the kind of birth they want are taken into account.

The WHO report comments:

> While most countries in the European Region have legal mandates for services during birth, in most cases the mandates are limited to the structures of the system: hospital buildings, hospital staff, equipment, organization. Five of the 24 countries in the survey do guarantee the woman the legal right to professional assistance during childbirth. . . .
>
> There is a trend in most countries . . . to use larger hospitals for birth. . . . So while attempts are being made everywhere in Europe to enlarge and strengthen the primary care component of health services and reduce the secondary and tertiary components, birth services are moving in the opposite direction. In three countries, this trend has reached the level where 35–50% of all births are in hospitals where there are over 5000 births annually. Only a few countries have official laws or regulations guaranteeing the woman the choice of place where she will give birth. Nevertheless, many countries (including some that guarantee choice of place) go to great lengths to discourage home births: regulations that pay the services for institu-

Table 13   Recommended and Actual Number of Visits for Uncomplicated Pregnancies

	3–5	6–7	8–11	12–15	16+	No recommendation
Recommended number of visits	3–5	6–7	8–11	12–15	16+	No recommendation
Number of countries	4	1	8	7	1	2
Actual number of visits	3–5	6–7	8–11	12–15	16	No information
Number of countries	5	3	3	3	1	8

Source: WHO, 1985.

Table 14   Screening During Pregnancy in 24 Countries

Procedure or condition screened for	Number of countries where screening is:			
	Routine	Selective	Not performed	No answer
Blood group	21	1	0	2
Toxoplasmosis	3	14	4	3
Rubella	8	13	1	2
Tetanus	1	7	14	2
Syphilus	5	19	0	0
Amniocentesis	0	22	0	2
Ultrasound	3	19	0	2

Source: WHO, 1985.

tional birth but not home birth; prosecution of midwives assisting home births; prosecution of couples having a home birth; withdrawal of professional care for home birth; threats to physicians who support home birth. The result is that the frequency of home birth in almost all developed European countries is less than 5%. . . .

The rapid increase in the technology used during birth has changed the clinical skills of both physicians and midwives. In one country, a study of the causes of the increasing Caesarean section rate found that one of the main contributors was physician training. It was found that there was little or no training in auscultation by stethoscope during labour; manipulation of the baby in the breech position through the wall of the mother's uterus to turn it so that its head points downwards; vaginal breech birth. . . . By contrast, training in the use of electronic fetal monitoring, ultrasound monitoring and scalp sampling was extensive.

Midwife skills are similarly shifting toward more competence with technology at the expense of clinical skills involving direct patient contact. Midwives have always been skillful at evaluating during labour the quality of the fetal heart tones as well as the rate, a skill that is invaluable in differentiating between fetal stress and fetal distress. With the advent of the electronic fetal monitor, this skill is being lost. The midwife sometimes no longer sits with the woman in labour but at a desk monitoring one or more electronic fetal monitors. . . . As more births take place in hospitals, midwives (like physicians) have become more and more afraid of assisting at a home birth. As a consequence, many midwives are becoming more like physicians in their style of care as well as their skills, and the complementary close personal social support and advocate role of midwives is disappearing.

Between 20 percent and 80 percent of women having babies in the developed world today describe themselves as having great difficulty in looking after the baby, and as feeling unhappy, tired, and unable to get things done. Everything seems like too much effort. When the baby is crying, they feel desperate and sometimes quite angry with the baby who has got them into this situation. However, everyone considers it normal to cry on the fifth day and to feel

Table 15 Incidence Rates (%) of Specified Procedures for Operative Delivery in Some European Countries

Country	Forceps (a)	Vacuum (b)	Caesarean section (c)	Operative vaginal (a + b)	Procedure[a] Total interventions (a + b + c)	Year	Source
Belgium	nr	nr	7.2	nr	a + b + 7.2	1979	Social Security statistics—incomplete
Czechoslovakia	1.3	1.0	4.0	2.3	6.3	1979	Hospital reports to Ministry of Health
Denmark	0.7	8.6	10.3	9.3	19.6	1979	Total birth survey—Ministry of Health
Finland	0.3	3.4	11.9	3.7	14.6	1979	Collected reports from Nat. Health Centre
France	8.0	4.0	8.0	12.0	20.0	1976	Representative sample—4600 births
Hungary	0.4	2.0	8.0	2.4	10.4		Annual report from obst. departments
Netherlands	1.7	3.6	3.6	5.3	8.9	1978	Ministry of Health—national data
Norway	3.2	3.4	8.0	6.6	14.6	1979	Medical birth registry—covers all births
Poland	0.8	0.4	5.0	1.2	6.2		National statistics
Rumania	nr	nr	4.6	nr	a + b + 4.6		National statistics
Sweden	0.3	6.8	11.7	7.1	18.8	1979	National medical birth registry—all births
UK:							
England & Wales	13.3	nr	7.3	13.3 + b	20.6 + b	1978	National survey—10% sample of hospital records
Scotland	13.0	nr	10.7	13.0 + b	23.7 + b	1978	National data—single births only

[a] nr = not reported.

Source: Phaff, J. M. L., ed. *Perinatal health services in Europe: Searching for better childbirth.* London, Croom Helm, 1986. ©1986 The Regional Office for Europe of the World Health Organization.

Table 16 Women's Choice in Selected Routine Procedures in Uncomplicated Births in Official Services in 23 Survey Countries

Procedure	Number of countries offering:	
	Choice	No choice
Shaving	5	18
Birth method	0	23
Birth position	3	20
Anesthesia/analgesia	10	13
People present	10	13
Choice of doctor	8	15
Holding dead newborn	11	12
Electronic fetal monitoring	5	18
Episiotomy	1	22

Source: WHO, 1985.

exhausted after the birth. In fact, this should rather be seen as a normal, healthy reaction on the part of the mother to her treatment during birth. What kind of society is this that creates these kinds of services for birth, subjecting the great human event of childbirth to this most unnatural discipline?

BIRTH IN CONTEXT

It has become commonplace to observe that childbirth is never natural but always influenced by cultural customs and rules. As a Danish midwife recalled, "A woman who had given birth at home without any kind of professional help said, 'My delivery. Well, is there really anything to talk about? The child wants to get out, and so you deliver it. Then, the day after, you know you've got diapers to wash.' I must have looked rather surprised. She then added, 'Every-

Table 17 Bonding Procedures at Birth in Official Services in 24 Survey Countries

Bonding procedure	Number of countries allowing procedure:	
	Yes	No
Infant placed on mother's abdomen at birth	7	17
Breast offered to infant in birth room	7	17
Mother/infant time together in birth room	13	11

Source: WHO, 1985.

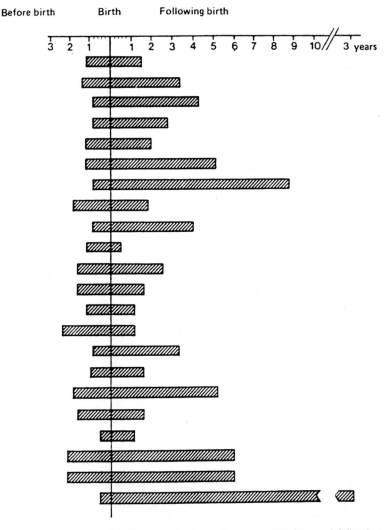

Figure 21 Duration of paid maternity leave (in months) before and following birth in 22 survey countries. (From WHO, 1985.)

thing else is something we make up.' '' According to social anthropologist Brigitte Jordan, ''childbirth is an intimate and complex transaction whose topic is physiological and whose language is cultural. Topic and language or, to put it another way, content and organization are never available one without the other.''

So the distinction between what is biological and what is social is in the realm of theory only. Instead, it makes sense to talk of childbirth as a *biosocial event,* uniting a universal physiological function with its culture-specific social matrix.

Thus, variations exist between cultures in the way they see and pattern birth, but the range within each culture is relatively narrow. There are, however, some general similarities across the world. Childbirth is universally seen as an important, often traumatic, event. Rules for managing this key event are needed: where, by whom, with whom, and how. It is too dangerous an event to be left to chance. Furthermore, each culture tends to regard its own way of managing childbirth as the only correct one. In her book *Birth in Four Cultures: A Cross-Cultural Investigation of Childbirth in Yucatan, Holland, Sweden, and the United States,* Brigitte Jordan frequently found people in one country asking her with an attitude of disbelief about the ridiculous, barbaric, unnecessary practices found in another.

> Thus Dutch midwives asked me (in a tone that said: Tell me I'm wrong), "Do they really do episiotomies on all women in the United States?"; Swedish midwives wanted to know why American obstetricians still use outmoded forceps when, in their view, vacuum extractors are much safer, and an eminent Swedish obstetrician considered differential care depending on ability to pay "an obscenity." American doctors often questioned me about the "backward" practices of the Indians, while the Indians, in turn, spoke only with moral indignation of such standard hospital procedures as vaginal examinations, episiotomies and the feet-in-stirrups position.

Each culture views its own birthing system as morally superior. This contains an important lesson to be applied to some of the material reviewed in this book. In the industrialized world, as we have seen, the dominant cultural definition of birth is a medical one; this is the context within which midwives today struggle to provide care for childbearing women. It follows from the medical definition of birth that obstetric practices are justified on medical and scientific grounds, whereas in other cultures such practices might be alternatively justified on the basis of family resources, appeals to nature to take its course, or the need to protect mother and child from damage by the supernatural: gods, dead family members, witches, and the like. Yet although medical practitioners in the industrialized world justify their practices by maintaining their scientific validity, this justification is in terms of knowing rather than being able to prove that this is the case. Often, scientific evidence just does not exist, and if it does, it may be far from clear-cut.

Much anthropological work, including Jordan's analysis, highlights the importance of the overall perspective on birth found in each culture. Is childbirth seen as a normal part of life, an inherently straightforward event? Or is it viewed as a form of illness, with a probably pathological outcome? Are women seen as the deliverers of their own babies, or as passive subjects to be delivered by others? The overall view has important implications for the type of care that is offered. For example, the Dutch notion of childbirth as a natural process precludes the use of drugs for women who, given the same conditions, would be provided with routine medication in the United States.

Cultural blindness is an important phenomenon. In 1877, a North American physician, Dr. Engelmann, was working on his collection of ancient Peruvian pottery when he heard about a funeral urn that had been found in some ancient Peruvian graves. The urn was in the possession of a Dr. Coates of Chester, Pennsylvania, and it was said to depict a typical Peruvian birth scene. When Dr. Engelmann finally got to see the urn some two years later, he was amazed to find the laboring woman shown in an upright position supported from behind by another woman. This was quite counter to the prevailing North American practice and led Dr. Engelmann to conduct extensive research into the cross-cultural evidence concerning position in labor (culminating in a book, *Labor among Primitive Peoples,* published in 1883). In a more recent anthropological endeavor, the late anthropologist Margaret Mead recounts how, on returning from New Guinea in the 1950s and reporting that women who had never borne children were able to lactate, she was challenged with skepticism and denial from North American doctors. Yet, of course, Mead's observations concerning this phenomenon were proved to the extent that there is now a considerable literature advising adoptive mothers how to stimulate lactation.

BIRTH SCENES

To paint a fuller picture of how childbirth is happening today, we give below three descriptions of births as they actually happened in 1986.

In the first of these scenes, the mother giving birth is having her first child in a Copenhagen hospital. She is twenty-five years of age and unemployed. Her labor lasts twelve hours and twenty minutes. Her midwife is also from Copenhagen. She is a direct-entry midwife, doing about 100 deliveries a year. She is thirty-eight years of age and has two children of her own.

Birth Scene 1

The mother has been sitting in the living room off the delivery ward, smoking. Then she goes into the room where her baby will be born and lies on the bed.

> *Woman:* My back hurts.
> The woman is shivering and has pains in her fingers.
> *Woman:* No—it's exhausting.
> The midwife washes her with a wet cloth. The woman smiles.
> *Woman:* No, it's too cold. There's a contraction coming. Hell, it hurts!
> *Midwife:* Breathe in the right way.

Woman: No, I can't.

The woman is sitting on the edge of the bed. She puts her arms around the midwife's neck and then gets down on the floor.

Woman: Now I'm down.

Midwife: Isn't it nice?

Woman: Yes.

The woman stands at the edge of the bed. The midwife is behind her, massaging her back.

Woman: If only something would happen! It's pushing into my stomach.

Midwife: As if you want to go to the toilet?

Woman: Yes. If only it didn't hurt so much!

The woman gets back onto the bed.

Midwife: We'll take a couple of contractions here now.

Woman: Oh!

The woman holds the midwife by the hand.

Woman: Oh, that was good.

The midwife wipes her face with a wet cloth.

Midwife: What are you feeling? Tell me. You know why it hurts—don't you?

Woman: I want to lie down.

Midwife: Let's take the next one.

The woman gets on the bed and has a contraction. Her arm is around the midwife's neck, so that the two of them are face to face.

Woman: If only it was all over. Hell, how it hurts!

She kicks angrily with one foot. The midwife strokes her hair.

Woman: When will this be over?

Midwife: Next time I'll give you the mask.

Woman: No!

Midwife: You can try it in the break between contractions. Did you do that the last time you delivered?

Woman: Yes.

Midwife: Just try it.

Woman: No, I don't want to.

She holds the midwife's hand.

Woman: I want this to be over. Oh no!

She shakes.

Midwife: Do you need to pee?

She examines the woman's lower abdomen.

Midwife: You've got a full bladder.

The woman sits on a bedpan.

Woman: Oh—no—hell! I can't pee.

She gets off. The midwife massages her back. The contractions are getting weaker.

Midwife: Now you should sit in the beanbag.

Woman: No!

She cries.

Midwife: Come on. But first I'd better do an internal examination.

The examination shows that the baby's head isn't in the right position.
Midwife: Now you'll have to lie down in the beanbag in a certain way.
Woman: Why?
Midwife: Because the head needs to get into the right position for the birth.
Woman: Ah!
Midwife: Lie on your knees and elbows, even though it sounds strange, then your contractions will get better.
Woman: They're good enough!
Midwife: I mean less painful.
Woman: Oh.
The woman lies on her knees over the beanbag pillow and moves her bottom from side to side.
Woman: Oh—ah—oh!
She lies on her side.
Woman: Hell, it hurts!
The midwife puts her hand on the woman's back.
Woman: Oh, I'm so tired!
She wants to push. The midwife leaves the room. After five minutes, she comes back.
Midwife: Let me examine you.
Woman: On, I'm going to sleep and sleep forever when this is over!
Midwife: The contractions aren't very good. Maybe we should use a drip.[1]
Woman: No!
She cries.
Midwife: Oh yes.
Woman: No!
A nurse comes in with a drip.
Midwife: Yes, this will help. You need to have this over and done with. I think we should listen to the baby's heart, and I want to put an electrode on the baby's head.
Woman: But then I won't be able to get up and walk.
Midwife: You're not supposed to do that anyway. You should stay in bed now!
She puts the electrode on.
Woman: Oh, it hurts so much!
Midwife: Yes, that's why we want to help you to get it over and done with. I'll put the light on.
The woman is on her side, panting. The midwife massages her back and holds her hand. The woman is on her back in the beanbag. She cries very unhappily. The electrode doesn't work. A new machine is brought into the room. The external monitor is put on.
Woman: Oh no!
She half sits up in the beanbag and pushes. The monitor is removed. The midwife performs an internal examination.
Midwife: Try to push next time—take hold of your legs. Bend your neck forward.

---

[1]Intravenous drugs to speed up labor.

The woman's legs are in stirrups. The midwife changes the delivery bed, shortening it by removing the end.

Midwife: Press! Push! Call the doctor.

A girl is born.

Woman: Oh—she's sweet—it's a girl.

The midwife puts the baby on the mother's stomach.

Woman: She's so tiny.

The midwife cuts the cord. The baby and the mother remain together for forty-five minutes. Then the doctor comes in to examine them.

Birth Scene 2

The second birth scene is a home birth in Denmark. The mother is forty-two years of age and is having her second child. Labor lasts seven hours and forty minutes. Her midwife, who is forty-four years of age and has three children, trained by direct entry. She does about sixty births a year, including twenty at home. She and the mother know each other quite well. Also present during the labor is one of the mother's friends, a relaxation class teacher, and an observing midwife. The room is lit only by candlelight.

The woman is having a bath. She sits up in the bathtub and washes all over. The midwife is in the bathroom helping her. She kneels down beside the woman. The friend walks around with the two-year-old son, trying to persuade him to go to bed.

Midwife: Does that feel good?

Woman: Yes. Is he asleep?

Friend: He's all right.

Woman: I can't deal with him now. God, it's bad; I've never had pain like this before.

The midwife massages her all over with soap.

Woman: So many people—babies—are born! This is the last time I'm going to give birth.

The midwife puts her hand on the woman's back.

Woman: Do you think I should stand up?

The woman drinks a mixture of homeopathic medicine: pulsatilla and belladonna. She then gets out of the bath and dries herself. The midwife massages her back. The woman moans, then showers again and dries herself.

Midwife: I'd like to examine you, and perhaps break your waters. I know that you'd rather I didn't, but your cervix isn't very open yet, and you're bleeding a little too much.

Woman: Is it too much?

She goes into the living room and lies down on her side. The midwife speaks gently to her.

Woman: Am I bleeding too much?

Midwife: I don't know.

The friend reads to the son. The woman has a contraction.

Woman: No—No—No!

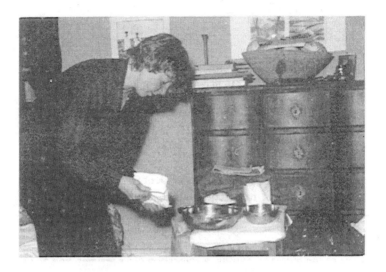

Figure 22 Preparing for birth.

Midwife: You're almost fully dilated! Do you want some water?

The woman drinks while the midwife examines her. She shivers and turns onto her side.

Woman: Hell, what a way to have guests!

Midwife: Hold on to me. Yes, you're pushing now.

The woman makes a long-drawn-out sound.

Midwife: You pushed! This time you can do what you want. Would you like to walk around or would you rather stay here? You decide.

Woman: I want to lie down here. Should I sit up, though?

Midwife: Try to sit up—just for a few contractions. That's good, that was a good push. Hold on to me.

Woman: I'm going to hurt you.

Midwife: No, you won't. Are you thirsty?

Woman: No.

The midwife listens to the baby's heart, which sounds good. She and the woman talk very quietly to each other. There is a long moaning sound. The midwife holds the woman's hand. Then silence.

Midwife: Relax your pelvis. Open your mouth, yes. Now push!

Woman: Eh, eh, ah!

The woman gets on her knees. The midwife is sitting in front of her on the floor, also on her knees. The woman puts her head on the midwife's shoulder, who then holds her head in her hands. They are finding a rhythm together.

The woman is now on all fours, moving forwards and backwards. The little boy is playing in the room; he goes over to his mother. The midwife talks to him.

Midwife: You should go to sleep now. (*To the woman.*) Does he bother you?

The woman sits straight with closed eyes. The midwife is next to her, hand on stomach. She listens to the heartbeat.

Midwife: The baby's fine, but needs to come out soon. Do you feel it moving down at all?

Woman: No, I don't feel anything like that.

The midwife dries her forehead. The woman moves forwards and backwards and pushes a little. The waters break. The woman closes her eyes, tries to lie down, and then get up again and half sits, naked. There is very little bleeding.

Woman: No, I can't.

She is disturbed because her son is there. The midwife is lying behind her, pressing into her back.

Woman: I can't. I don't want to—no, I can't!

The midwife continues to massage her back while listening to the baby's heartbeat.

Midwife: It's all right.

There's a contraction. She lies on her side with her eyes closed.

Woman: There's really a long time between contractions now. What happens if I don't have any more? It's irritating me. I just can't.

She pushes.

Midwife: Only push when there's a contraction. Follow the body's urge to push.

Woman: If only I could go to sleep; then you could go home. If only you could do something.

She pushes suddenly. There's another contraction. The midwife listens to the heart. She examines the mother again. Then a boy is born.

The observing midwife notes, "For the last hour, I was sitting behind the mother and she was leaning on me. I couldn't write anything at this stage; just sitting there seemed much more important. I was very tired, but I felt I had to support her, too. Finally, just before the birth, her friend succeeded in getting her son to sleep, so the four of us women were together for the last fantastic, and very quiet, hour. When the baby was born, we realized that the light of dawn was streaming in through the window. The mother was very tired after the birth, but she still held the baby all the time."

Birth Scene 3

The third mother is having her baby in a county general hospital in Denmark. Her midwife is thirty-two years of age with no children. She trained in England. She does about 100 deliveries a year. The mother is a thirty-year-old physiotherapist, and it is her first child. Her labor lasts sixteen hours and ten minutes. The woman's husband is present.

The woman is standing, bending over the end of the bed, breathing deeply. Her husband is massaging her.

Midwife: Do you like standing like that?

The midwife is standing next to the woman, wiping her face with a wet cloth.

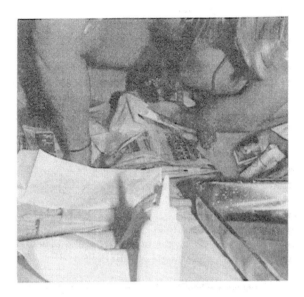

Figure 23   The birth.

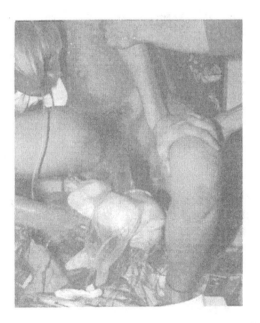

Figure 24   A boy.

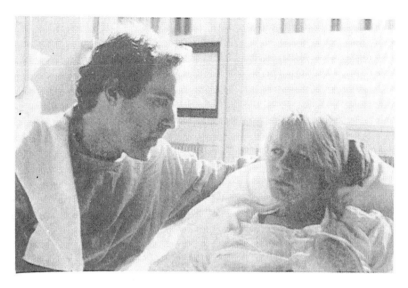

Figure 25 Breathing together.

Midwife: When were you examined last?

Woman: At two o'clock or a little later—my cervix was five centimeters dilated then.

Midwife: I'd like to examine you again to see how far on you are, so could you go back to the bed, please?

Woman: Yes.

She climbs into bed and lies on her side; then she tries to turn on her back, gets a contraction, turns on her side again, and then repeats the whole process. The midwife waits patiently for her to lie on her back. At last she is able to examine the woman.

Midwife: You're six centimeters now.

Woman: Not more?

Midwife: That's not bad; it's a good sign. The baby's head is quite far down. Do you want to stay in bed?

Woman: Yes.

She turns on her side, and the midwife places a pillow between her legs. Between contractions, the midwife wipes her face.

Midwife: I don't want to rupture your membranes; they protect the baby, and the contractions aren't that strong yet. Do you want something to drink?

Woman: Yes, thanks.

Midwife: If you think the contractions are too tough, you're welcome to use the mask.[2] It won't make the pain go completely, but it will take the edge off it.

Woman: I'll probably need it soon.

---

[2]To breathe a pain killer.

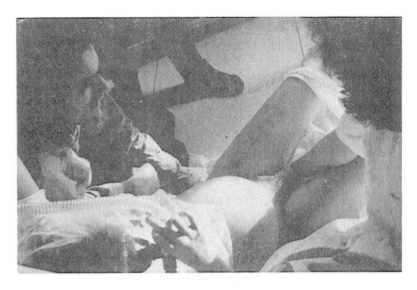

Figure 26 Halfway through the labor.

The woman is breathing deeply during each contraction. There are pearls of sweat on her upper lip. The midwife goes to get a cold drink for both parents.

The midwife listens to the baby's heart between contractions. The woman drinks.

Midwife: I think it's a boy—the heart rate is 120; girls are usually 130–160.

Father: It's a boy; I knew it!

The woman breathes deeply.

Woman: I want to try the mask.

The woman takes it and breathes deeply into it.

Midwife: I'm going to examine you again, and then I might rupture the membranes to help the baby on its way.

She examines the woman again, washes her, puts her on a bedpan, and cuts her pubic hair. The woman continues to take gulps of air from the mask.

The midwife ruptures the membranes; the waters are brownish-green.

Midwife: I think I'll put an electrode on the baby's head.

She attaches it.

Midwife: The waters were slightly greenish, so I want to check the heart rate.

Father: I noticed that, too.

Woman: That's okay.

The woman is still on her back—on the bedpan. She then gets off the bedpan and moves onto her side, using the mask half the time.

Midwife: Tell me if you want to push.

During each contraction, the midwife gently caresses the woman's stomach. The woman is very introverted and quiet, clinging to the mask. The midwife puts a pillow between her knees.

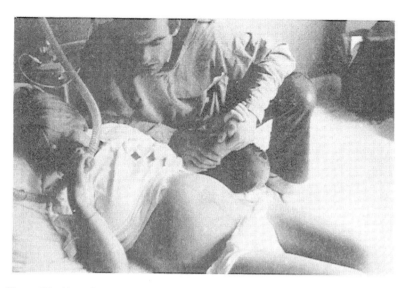

Figure 27 Use of the mask.

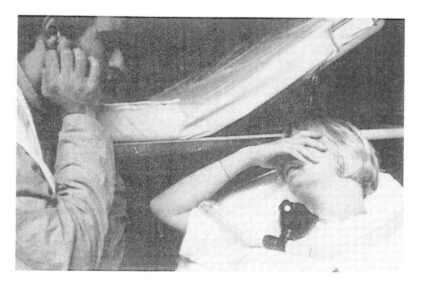

Figure 28 "Help me!"

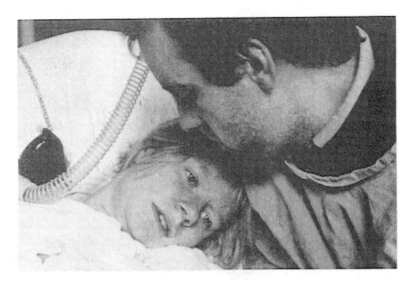

Figure 29   "I am not going to make it!"

Midwife: Would you like to put your legs into the stirrups if I put them down low?

Woman: Yes, I could do that.

The midwife leans against her right knee.

Woman: Now I'm having a contraction.

Midwife: Good, now push like I told you. That's right—you are clever! Elbows to the side—very good. Now I can see a bit of the head. (*To the husband.*) Look!

The woman continues to push and do as she's told.

Midwife: Now, this is better. Push like you're going to the toilet. That's fine, very, very good. I think I'm going to give you some anesthesia. It's getting a bit unpleasant now, isn't it? But you're doing very well.

She has to push the baby's head back so as to give the injection (a pudendal block).

Midwife: Now something's happening. Do you want to look in the mirror?

Woman: Well—yes.

She smiles politely. The midwife moves the bed and arranges the mirror.

Midwife: See!

Woman: Yes.

Her head is on one side, her eyes closed.

Midwife: Can you see?

Woman: Yes.

Her eyes are still closed. A young doctor comes in. He looks confused. The midwife cuts the perineum with scissors. When the baby's head is born, she suctions it.

Midwife: Oh—the baby's already crying; it can't wait to get out. Now hold the baby.

Woman: No, I don't know.

Midwife: Yes, come on; you'll be glad afterwards. Come—hold it and tell us what sex it is.

The woman holds the half-born baby and, together with the midwife, draws it out and lifts it onto her stomach.

Midwife: Now—what is it?

Woman: A boy—hello, Martin!

She tries to look at the baby, but her position makes it awkward, so she touches the baby as it lies on her stomach.

Midwife: I'm going to give your stomach a little push to get the placenta out.

The woman is looking at the baby and her husband, smiling. The father is waiting for the placenta to be born.

Midwife: Do you want to see the placenta?

Woman: Yes.

She takes the placenta and shows it to the woman.

Midwife: This is what was up inside your uterus.

Woman: It's big!

Midwife: Can you imagine how big the scar there would be if the uterus didn't contract itself? Now, here are the membranes in which the baby was lying—and here is what he's been looking at—it looks like a tree—isn't it beautiful?

Woman: That's fantastic.

She smiles politely, then holds the baby close to her face, looking at him.

Midwife: Now I'm going to wash you and stitch you up—I had to cut you.

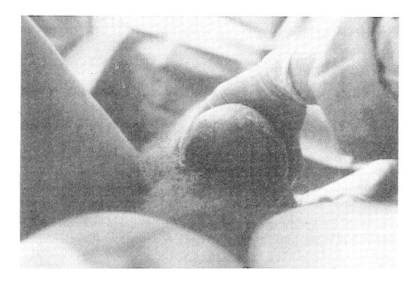

Figure 30   The birth.

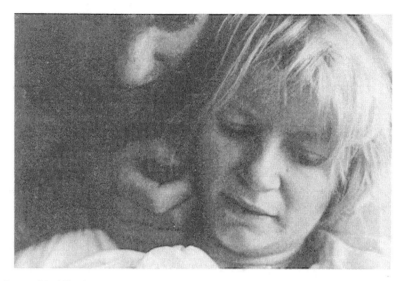

Figure 31   Wonder.

Woman: Oh, I didn't notice that.

Midwife: No, you're anesthetized, that's why.

For the next thirty minutes, the midwife sutures the woman. The doctor takes the baby and examines him. The baby cries, and everybody laughs.

Doctor: It's nice to hear his voice.

The baby is put to the mother's breast. Then he's weighed, dressed, and given to the father to hold.

BIRTH AS LIBERATION[3]

When writing about childbirth, and the position of midwives today, it is all too easy to emphasize only the negative aspects. Midwives are having a difficult time, birth is being changed by technology, and women as mothers are defined by the obstetrical and social establishment. In the birth scenes described in this chapter, these themes are certainly present. It is clear, for example, that giving birth in a hospital makes it easier for the midwife to use technology—to speed up labor, to attach a monitor, to offer the mother pain relief. Yet this is only one side of the coin. Wherever it happens, childbirth can be a positive experience, and the task of the midwife can be a supportive and joyful one. Noticeable in all the accounts presented here is the midwife's sensitivity to what the mother is

[3]This is an edited translation of part of the book, *Twelve Planned Homebirths in Storströms County in Denmark,* by J. Moeller, S. Houd, U. Marcussen, D. Gannik, and H. Wulf (Copenhagen: Graficus, 1982).

feeling—not only how her uterus is behaving and the extent to which she feels and minds the pain, but smaller things, such as whether she feels tired or thirsty or has become stuck in an uncomfortable position. The midwife is with the woman, interpreting her condition, mediating between her and her environment. As one Danish midwife has said:

> The job of the midwife is to assist with the physical side of the birth, but she can also help birth to be a psychological birth for the mother and her partner. In order to do this, the midwife must help the woman and the family to participate actively in the birth and to take responsibility for what's happening. On the very deepest level, the experience of birth may be an experience of rebirth. Some women say when they give birth that they feel it to be a mysterious or religious experience, they feel "connected with earth and eternity", they understand "the meaning of life" or are suddenly able to see it as "part of a greater whole". On the level of the woman's personality, she may find new strengths in herself as she "gives" birth. And on the level of social experiences, birth can be a positive and integrative experience for a family.
>
> When birth happens in an institution it's difficult for these things to happen. Most of the woman's energy tends to get used up in the effort of living up to the expectations of the institution. The midwife works an 8-hour shift, taking over from another midwife whatever point in the labouring/birthing process has been reached. There are fetal monitors and resuscitation equipment in the birth room, tiles on the walls; the midwife's wearing a white, synthetic dress or a blue uniform, or whatever, and probably a cap as well. How does this make her feel? How does it make the mother feel?
>
> Perhaps we're just as afraid of the ecstatic element in birth as we are of its pain and discomfort, with the result that we need to suppress the possibility of ecstasy by institutionalizing birth in this hygienic and mechanistic way.

A large American collective, The Farm in Tennessee, developed the practice of handling deliveries in accordance with a semireligious philosophy. This places birth in a context that enables the ecstatic aspects of birth to be experienced. The community itself was established in 1972 with a population of 1500. Lay midwifery among Farm members began with three deliveries in a caravan and subsequently expanded to become a comprehensive alternative to official care, taking in clients from outside the community. On The Farm, it is usual for deliveries to take place in the home. There is always at least one midwife present. New midwives are trained by accompanying the experienced midwives (a return to the premodern tradition discussed in Chapter 3). As Ina May Gaskin describes it in her book *Spiritual Midwifery,* Farm midwives work to create an expectant atmosphere around the delivery that makes it possible for this to be an experience of culmination for all those present. The "pregnant couple" are encouraged to work at their mutual relationship, and during the delivery it is common for them to have close physical contact with one another.

The contractions are described as rushes of energy, and the woman is encouraged to show courage and veneration toward the forces of nature, reflected in the delivery. The spiritual side of the experience is emphasized through the concentration on the reception of the new child by all those present. At the physical level, this is demonstrated by several people holding the child's head when it is being born.

Behind such practices and observations, there is a core idea of some importance to the midwife's work: the idea of birth as a therapeutic process. During birth, many women confront, live through, and integrate various repressed painful experiences of their own. The midwife's task is to help the mother to do this. She acts as a therapist, encouraging the mother openly to express the whole spectrum of feelings she may have during childbirth: fear, pain, panic, anger, joy, and ecstasy.

For one of these feelings—pain—there exists a particular repertoire of cultural responses that midwives encounter daily in their work, whether at home or in the hospital. It is part of the medical model of birth that pain should be pharmacologically relieved. Drugs are given for the pain of illness, goes the argument, so they should also be given for the pain of birth.

The difficulty with this is that pain and ecstasy at birth may be closely interrelated. Some women experience the pain of birth as violent, and birth is felt and remembered as a chaotic and destructive process. Others are given pain relief that relieves not only the pain but also the possibility of ecstasy. The pain of childbirth is poorly understood. To consider it in some sense a meaningful pain is not to say that all women should suffer in childbirth, but it is important to point out that through the experience of pain in birth a woman's consciousness may be altered in significant and subtle ways. It is theoretically possible, for example, that the experience of pain enables a degree of preparation for the child, which makes its sex less important than it might otherwise be. When women talk about the pain of labor, it is common to hear them say, "Yes, it hurts, but you forget that as soon as the baby's born and you hold it in your arms."

As Jordan notes in *Birth in Four Cultures,* while some women appear to give birth without experiencing pain, pain is a recognized and expected part of the birth process in almost all societies. The idea that primitive women give birth easily and without pain is fallacious. "What is of interest . . . however, is not whether women do or do not experience pain, but rather what sort of an object pain becomes in different systems, whether it is highlighted or discounted, what kinds of occasions its occurrence provides for displaying the nature of the system, and so on."

Midwives encounter the fear and pain of women in labor and need to confront these emotions in themselves. If this is not done, they may project their own feelings onto the laboring woman. Some midwives shut themselves off from the experience of pain and prefer to use pain relief as much as possible. Others feel that if they establish a good relationship with the woman, they may be able to do something about her need for pain relief by supporting her and by lessening her perception of the pain itself. Touching and massage can be valuable aids. These have a physiological component, because pressure and touch can subdue the pain transfer between nerve cells in the body.

Sometimes it happens that, during the delivery, the woman regresses to a manner of expressing herself that is not accepted in the grown-up world. Some midwives are aware that such regressions can be a starting point for women to work on repressed feelings in relation to independence and authority. Women may scream or say things they would not say in everyday life. Screams can be liberating. Thus, Janov made the scream a cornerstone in his therapeutic treatment, primal therapy.

It can be equally important for the midwife not to let herself be carried away by the expressions of the woman in labor. She needs to be capable of meeting the mother with a mixture of empathetic understanding and calm authority.

When the midwife and the woman in labor have this kind of bond with each other, problems may arise that can be compared to what are called in psychoanalysis transference problems. The midwife/therapist is regarded as a parent figure, and the woman displays childish reactions toward her. Another problem is that the mother/person in treatment might fall in love with the midwife/therapist, regarding her/him with a childish love and devotion. Both successful childbirth and successful therapy should result in adult relationships between the two participants in the interaction. Sometimes, the midwife needs to work further on her relationship to the woman in labor after the birth. The midwife must climb down from her pedestal and become a human being.

Birth exposes the position of the midwife in several ways. In itself, it is a drama about life and death. The midwife is congratulated and surrounded with happiness when everything goes well—but she also is blamed if something has gone wrong. Many midwives develop extensive defense mechanisms to protect themselves from this intrinsic vulnerability. Some of these are:

- *denial,* in which the midwife denies to herself that fear has any place at all in a modern delivery, so she intervenes quickly and starts controlling the birth
- *projection,* in which the midwife projects her own experience of fear on the woman in labor (if the woman in labor refuses to submit to the fear of the midwife and its consequences, she may easily be met with the anger of the midwife)
- *rationalization,* in which the delivery process is understood solely as a medical matter and fear is camouflaged in medical terms and technology
- *compensation,* in which the midwife takes over the situation of the woman in labor by telling the woman what she feels before the woman herself has been able to develop her own perception of the situation

- *reaction formation,* in which the midwife loves her work blindly and refuses to acknowledge its controversial side (such a midwife may have an idealized and sentimental attitude toward the woman in labor)

One implication of the midwife's vulnerability is that midwives need their own support systems, and perhaps expert therapeutic help, to understand and work through their experiences of assisting women during childbirth. They need to talk about fear and insecurity—for example, in connection with responsibility and the risk of being accused of having made a mistake. This is difficult in the hierarchical system of the hospital.

Aside from its implications for the midwife's role, the idea of the liberating possibility of birth also implies that women play an active role in delivering their own children. In her study of women having their first babies, Dana Breen (1975) found that the women who managed best as mothers were those who scored as masculine on a test designed to distinguish between masculine and feminine qualities. Breen concluded that the cultural norm equating femaleness with passivity and maleness with activity is inappropriate when speaking of adjustment to motherhood. There are many other research findings showing how a feeling of control, expressed in the mother's conviction that she did indeed deliver her own child, aids both her mental and physical health after childbirth. However, the issue is complex. This seems to be an area in which class differences exist and may be an expression of different priorities in giving birth. Some studies have shown that working-class women welcome those childbirth technologies they see as making delivery a faster and more comfortable experience for them, so long as the baby's health is not jeopardized.

Chapter Five

Protest

As we have seen, health services for childbirth today are in disarray. The changes in the organization and content of maternity services that have taken place in Europe over the past thirty years are being subjected to a new critical scrutiny. The staffing of maternity services is seen to raise fundamental questions about the needs of mothers, babies, and families and about who is best able to meet those needs. This is one context within which today's debate about the role of the midwife is carried on: What is wrong with the official health services for pregnancy and birth, and where does the midwife stand as the expert in normal processes?

Another, broader context for this debate is the modern critique of medical care. In the period since World War II, a number of factors have coincided to give birth to an organized movement of health care users who have protested against their powerless and infantilized role within the official health care system. They have questioned some basic precepts of that system, including its dependence on a medical model of health and its resort to high technology, high cost solutions. The subject of perinatal care has been a focus of this protest. Pregnancy and birth are the best examples of the medicalization of life, the conversion of normal physiological experiences into the subject and treatment matter of professional medicine. At the opposite end of life, the same thing has happened to death. Birth provides a unique example of the long-term biosocial process of child rearing and individual development, which can be damaged by the way in which it begins.

Today, a chorus of voices can be heard saying what is wrong and what needs to be done about the disarray of childbirth. Some themes rise clearly above the cacophony.

THE PROTESTING CONSUMER

Among the reasons for the rise of the consumer health movement is increasing public recognition that many health problems lie beyond the reach of medical science and technology. The improved general health of people in industrialized countries has caused a shift from acute to chronic illness; around 80 percent of all illness is now of the chronic variety. There has thus been an increase in health problems that cannot be effectively treated by drug therapies and other immediate physical interventions. As part of this picture, it is unfortunately true to say that, in countries such as the United Kingdom and the United States, medical care has not succeeded in curing social inequalities in health. In the United Kingdom, for example, perinatal mortality is considerably higher in families in social class V (lowest) than in those in social class I (highest), and similar differences obtain according to the mother's country of birth (Tables 18 and 19). The reasons for these inequalities are complex, but one message emerges clearly: professional medical care on its own is not the answer. There is no consistent relationship between levels of spending on formal health care in different countries and the mortality ratings of the countries. Table 20 shows the percentage of gross national product (GNP) devoted to health care in a number of countries in relation to their mortality ratings, here represented by the standardized mortality index, which goes from 1 (good) to 10 (bad). The country (Sweden) that has the best standardized mortality index spends the highest proportion of its GNP on formal health care, but the Federal Republic of Germany, which comes next in terms of the proportion of its GNP spent on formal health care, does worst in mortality terms.

A key factor behind the consumer health movement is the unproven scientific status or proven hazards of some medical care. According to the U.S. Office of Technology Assessment, around 90 percent of all medical care methods have not been established as efficacious and safe. Some 20 percent of illnesses occur as a result of medical treatment. At the same time, the escalating costs of medical care in many countries have added a cash crisis to the crisis of confidence in the ability of medical care to provide the goods—that is, health. David Banta, in a paper presented at the Joint International Conference on Appropriate Technology in Brazil in 1985, has said that:

Table 18   Perinatal Deaths by Social Class,
England and Wales, 1985

Social class[a]	Perinatal death rate[b]
I	7.8
II	7.5
III manual	8.8
III nonmanual	9.2
IV	11.1
V	12.4
All	9.8

[a]Legitimate births only, based on father's occupation.
[b]Per 100 total births.
Source: Office of Population Censuses and Surveys Monitors (DH3 87/3 and DH3 87/1 [1987]).

Table 19   Perinatal Deaths by Mother's Country of Birth,
England and Wales, 1985

Mother's country of birth	Perinatal death rate[a]
All	9.8
United Kingdom	9.5
Irish Republic	12.7
Australia, Canada, and New Zealand	10.1
New Commonwealth and Pakistan	12.7
New Commonwealth:	
India	10.1
Bangladesh	12.9
East Africa	10.8
West Africa	13.9
South and rest of Commonwealth Africa	11.6
West Indies	14.7
Malta, Gibraltar, Cyprus	6.8
Rest of New Commonwealth	7.9
Pakistan	17.9
Not stated or at sea	144.7
Rest of the world	8.5

[a]Per 100 total births.
Source: Office of Population Census and Surveys Monitors (DH3 87/3 and DH3 87/1 [1987]).

Medical technology, or the drugs, devices and medical and surgical procedures used in medical care, has been estimated to account for up to 50% of the increase in the cost of medical care. . . .

Perinatal technology raises additional problems. First, birth is a normal process, with a satisfactory result in the vast majority of cases without technological intervention. Second, two people are involved, the mother and the baby, and an intervention to help one may harm the other.

In addition to these broad problems of perinatal technology, questions have been raised about a number of obstetric technologies. A number of authors and scientists, including obstetricians, have criticized the routine obstetric procedures such as electronic fetal monitoring, Caesarean section, induction of labour, perineal shaving, episiotomy and obstetric anaesthesia. Some procedures, such as perineal shaving, have been called essentially useless. In most cases, however, this issue is one of risks versus benefits. For example, the risks of the widespread routine use of electronic fetal monitoring, such as infection and associated Caesarean sections, appear to outweigh the benefits.

Over the past ten to fifteen years, many perinatal procedures assumed to be scientifically effective have been shown not to be so. This is not the place to summarize this research, but a brief quotation from it is in order, since questions about technology and the place of birth in particular are constantly raised in discussing the present and future of midwifery.

In a 1983 review by Cynthia Fraser of the scientific basis of selected perinatal procedures, the following observations were made, taking account of the available evidence:

Table 20   Levels of Formal Health Care Spending and Mortality in 10 Countries

	Rank according to:	
Country	Percentage of GNP spent on formal health care	Standardized mortality index
Australia	6	5
Canada	7	6
France	5	7
Germany, Federal Republic of	2	10
Italy	9	8
Netherlands	4	2
Sweden	1	1
Switzerland	8	3
United Kingdom	10	4
United States	3	9

Source: Health and Disease. Open University, 1985.

The premise that an increase in the quantity of antenatal care for each pregnant woman will consequently lead to a decline in perinatal mortality rates has not been adequately demonstrated. Although an inverse correlative relationship has been shown to exist, a causal relationship has not been identified.

The trend towards hospitalization of births in the western world has been based on the assumption that hospitals are safer places for both mother and infant and, consequently, would lead to a decline in perinatal and maternal mortality rates. . . . While there has indeed been a fall in perinatal mortality, this does not imply that hospitalization and its accompanying technology is responsible.

There is a lack of evidence as to when and under what circumstances intervention is efficacious. What is known is that Caesarean section, like any other abdominal operation, carries a small risk of fatality for the mother and increases the risk of respiratory distress for the infant. . . . Instrumental deliveries carry the risk of intracranial haemorrhage and other body damage for the infant. There is uncertainty as to which type of instrumental delivery is preferable. . . . Better documentation of the benefits and hazards of interventionist delivery is required.

Since this review was published, the benefits and hazards of many standard perinatal procedures have been better documented. The (British) National Perinatal Epidemiology Unit/WHO *A Classified Bibliography of Controlled Trials in Perinatal Medicine 1940-1984* listed in 1985 more than 2500 trials evaluating such procedures. This sort of systematic work is necessary to test all accepted ideas of safety and effectiveness. Unfortunately, midwives have very limited opportunities to conduct this kind of research themselves, but two of the studies subjecting common procedures to the test of controlled experimentation were carried out by a midwife, Mona Romney.

In reexamining accepted notions of what is safe and valuable in perinatal care, the idea of appropriate technology has come to the fore as a useful way of looking at the relationship between technical procedures and health promotion. In 1984-86, the World Health Organization (WHO) held three conferences on the theme of appropriate perinatal technology: one in Washington, D.C., on the antenatal period, one in Brazil on birth, and one in Italy on the period following birth. These meetings produced many recommendations, including the following.

The prenatal period

The users of perinatal services should have informed choice with regard to their care options. . . .

The planning, the giving and the evaluation of prenatal care should involve at all levels the pregnant woman, companions including family, as well as the community. Consideration should be given to the central role of the pregnant and birthing woman in her own care. . . .

Continuity of care should be encouraged from the planning of pregnancy through care of the infant and family during the neonatal period. In their training, health care providers should be sensitized to the importance of continuity of care, and alternatives within existing systems should be developed that will provide continuity.

Prenatal care should be provided within the context of a primary health care system. . . .

Health care providers should provide prenatal care which includes appropriate psychosocial aspects, health promotion and health education, and the use of technology appropriate to individual settings. . . .

Before widespread use, a technology should be evaluated in terms of efficacy, safety, psychosocial effects, ethical consequences, social and economic cost, and the broader implications of its impact on the overall perinatal health care system.

Technologies already in use should be periodically evaluated according to the principles outlined above. The ethical and legal issues involved in such evaluation must be carefully assessed.

The use of a technology should be limited to indications in which it has been demonstrated to be effective.

Birth

Countries with some of the lowest perinatal mortality rates in the world have Caesarean section rates of less than 10%. There is no justification for any region to have a rate higher than 10–15%. . . .

There is no evidence that routine fetal monitoring has a positive effect on the outcome of pregnancy. Electronic fetal monitoring should be carried out only in carefully selected cases related to high perinatal mortality rates and where labour is induced. Research should investigate the selection of women who might benefit from fetal monitoring. Meanwhile, national health services should abstain from purchasing new equipment. . . .

There is no indication for shaving pubic hair nor for an enema before delivery.

It is not recommended that the pregnant woman be placed in a dorsal lithotomy position during labour and delivery. Walking should be encouraged during labour and each woman must freely decide which position to adopt during delivery.

The perineum should be protected wherever possible.

Systematic use of episiotomy is not justified.

The induction of labour should be reserved for specific medical indications. No region should have rates of induced labour higher than 10%.

During delivery, the routine administration of analgesic or anaesthetic drugs . . . should be avoided.

Artificial early rupture of membranes as a routine process is not justifiable.

The postpartum period

Poverty is the greatest threat to the health to the woman and the infant. In the absence of concerted measures to promote social equity, little improvement can be expected in maternal and infant mortality and morbidity. . . .

The structure of health care systems and the way they operate are influenced by commercial interests and by the needs and perspectives of professionals and others who work in them. When such influences are strong, they must be publicly recognized and, if necessary, controlled. . . .

Every woman and infant should have access to a basic level of care regardless of whether the birth takes place at home or in a primary or secondary health care setting. At every birth, wherever it takes place, one attendant should take overall responsibility for the woman and infant.

Government agencies should support the provision of health care by alternative providers, such as empirical midwives. The role and efficiency of these alternative providers should be systematically evaluated. . . .

Any technology used in postnatal or postpartum care should undergo evaluation before its introduction for general use. Such evaluation should include efficacy and safety, economic implications, and cultural acceptability.

The move against routine use of technology and in favor of such nontechnological items as continuity of care is obvious from these recommendations. Sometimes, the appropriate technology is not at all difficult to find. The most appropriate "technology" for childbirth is the mother. Hence the frequently heard medical saying that the best transport device for the fetus is the uterus. A WHO report called *Appropriate Technology for Thermal Control of Newborn Babies* gave the traditional practice of many cultures the status of a scientific recommendation in saying that healthy babies should stay in the mother's bed after delivery. Thus, the technology most needed is wider hospital beds to facilitate this practice. The use of the mother's body to warm and care for even low birth weight infants (the "kangaroo method") began to be promoted after reports from Colombia of its success (Figures 32 and 33).

At the same time as technology is questioned, health is increasingly coming to be seen as a resource that individuals and communities can, and indeed must, supply for themselves. The key concept is *self-help*. Central to the idea of self-help is a social model of how health is produced; it is not possible to explain or understand much health behavior except by reference to the social context of everyday life. Health may not be the highest priority in life for everyone. Risk-taking can be a rational and responsible way of acting; self-reliance is an expression of human dignity. Caring and coping are as important as and, in fact, intrinsic to curing.

Some self-help groups in perinatal and other fields have arisen not only in response to perceived deficiencies within the medical care system but also as

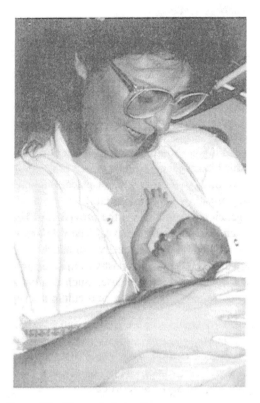

Figure 32 Closeness is healing.

ways of making up for a lack of social support within the social system. The development of the self-help movement has highlighted the absurdity of the term *consumer* as a description of health service users, for health system users often lack the ability to choose from a range of options, the very choice exercised by the consumer in the market place. Indeed, the professionalization of medicine means that many users of health services lack the information that would permit choice. How many mothers giving birth in Europe today, for example, know the statistics comparing the safety and effectiveness of midwives with those of obstetricians? Or the statistics comparing the safety of home and hospital birth? Or the outcomes of the controlled trials that have been done of increasing common technological procedures, such as ultrasound scanning and the use of electronic fetal monitors? Knowledge is power. Power is what users of medical care, including women having babies, generally do not have.

As we saw in Chapter 2, women's unique position as health care providers means they have a particular interest in the self-help movement. Over the past twenty years, the feminist movement has articulated a strong case for placing women's health care in women's hands. Reproductive care is the pivot of this protest. As Sheryl Ruzek (1979) wrote in her history, *The Women's Health Movement,* "While critics argue that the health system is oppressive and unresponsive to the needs of both men and women, feminists find it particularly problematic for women. First, the very organization of the health care system reflects and perpetuates the social ideology of women as sex objects and reproductive organs. In the promotion of the specialty of obstetrics and gynecology, women are encouraged to enter the health system through their reproductive organs."

Some years ago, groups such as the Boston Women's Health Collective met to discuss female knowledge of female bodies and the kinds of services women might want to fit in with this knowledge. At that time—the late 1960s—the movement for childbirth reform was already under way. Feminists were initially reluctant to become involved in childbirth issues, since there seemed to be more need for health care reforms that would enable women to dispense with their traditional reproductive burdens. The politics of abortion, day care, and so on dominated the early feminist health consciousness. However, soon the two movements—self-help and feminist—began to feed into one another. The demand for changes in childbirth practices became part of the demand for reform of health services for women so as to provide woman-oriented and woman-sensitive care (Figure 34).

Midwifery fits comfortably into this picture, for woman-sensitive care is what the midwife has traditionally provided. In providing care for normal preg-

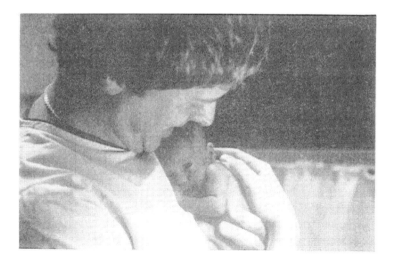

Figure 33 Getting to know each other.

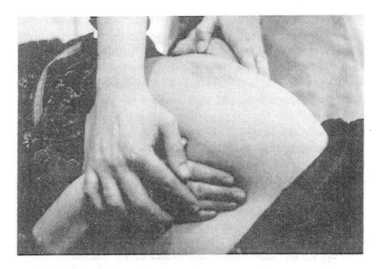

Figure 34   Self-help prenatal care.

nancies and births, she has encouraged or enabled women to take control for themselves of the process of giving birth. Midwives are not trained to specialize in interventions that remove the possibility of control from the mother. On the contrary, they are educated to see childbearing and childrearing as continuous processes in which the mother figures as an individual in her social context, not merely as a container for the uterus and the fetus. It is less easy to see how in practice midwives have been active in providing alternative woman-centered care. Constraints operate to reduce visibility: the illegality of midwifery in some places, for example, or the fact that the most radical midwives may be those who leave the official system and go underground, practicing forms of midwifery care that are undocumented and unacknowledged, except of course by the women who use them.

ALTERNATIVE PERINATAL SERVICES
IN EUROPE AND NORTH AMERICA

As part of a WHO survey of perinatal health services in Europe, in 1981 we researched the provision of what we call alternative perinatal services in ten countries (Canada, Denmark, France, Federal Republic of Germany, the Netherlands, Sweden, U.S.S.R., United Kingdom, United States, and Yugoslavia). Since alternative perinatal services by definition are not monitored by official systems of statistical data collection, the information for this study was not easy to collect. To gather data, we actually had to use the kind of informal social networks that play a key role in alternative health care.

In eight of the ten countries in our sample, we found alternative services both within and outside the official system of perinatal care. For the remaining two, both socialist countries, we had no evidence of similar services. In one of these two countries (U.S.S.R.), however, a decentralized structure of primary health care allowed a considerable flexibility among care providers in meeting the local needs of women having babies. In the second (Yugoslavia), it was interesting to note that the official services had incorporated several elements of traditional noninterventionist perinatal care in that region, including continuity of care and perineal massage with oil during the second stage of labor.

Despite differences between countries, two common themes emerged in the development of alternative perinatal services. These themes are the limitation of choice imposed on women having babies by the way in which the official services have developed in recent years, and the lack of attention paid within these services to the idea of pregnancy, childbirth, and parenthood as a continuous process embedded in the totality of human social life. In contrast, existing alternative services focus on the desire of childbearing women to choose a form of care appropriate to their personal needs. They also stress the nature of childbearing as a social rather than a purely medical event.

Eight of the study countries had a range of user organizations in the perinatal care field. One example is the Danish organization Parents and Childbirth, which has an eighteen-point agenda demonstrating the broad platform of many such organizations. Parents and Childbirth campaigns for:

- Exchange of experiences among parents
- Communication of parents' experiences to health professionals
- Formulation of delivery plans by parents
- Acceptance of such plans by care-givers
- Better social and financial conditions for parents, including longer postnatal leave for employed women
- Prenatal and postnatal classes for parents
- Parental choice about the place of delivery
- Alternative delivery positions
- Respect for the child's experience at birth
- Design of alternative apparatus for electronic fetal heart rate monitoring in labor (so that women in labor can move around freely), such apparatus not to be used routinely
- An undisturbed period of thirty to forty-five minutes just after birth for parent-child bonding
- The midwife who attended the birth to visit the mother at least once after the birth
- More counseling and information on breastfeeding
- Opportunities for employed mothers to breastfeed
- Free visiting in the postnatal wards
- Free parental visiting of hospitalized children

- More day care places for the children of employed parents
- Education for childbirth at school

This list makes no division between the narrow health care needs and wider social needs of parents. It emphasizes choice but is not inherently antitechnology. It favors the development of more appropriate technology.

Organizations of individuals working in alternative perinatal services usually begin at a local level and initially focus on a single theme or complaint to do with the way the official services function. We found that three themes were particularly likely to be prominent in the history of these organizations: (1) not enough choice as to place of delivery among service users; (2) bad hospital conditions for childbearing women; (3) overuse of technology in childbirth.

For example, Parents and Childbirth was set up because, in the early 1970s, some parents wanted to improve conditions in hospitals, and especially to make the father's presence at delivery an accepted practice. From this beginning, a Danish organization emerged, and special interest groups mushroomed, including a delivery position group and a home birth group.

Similar organizations in other countries have similar histories. In the United Kingdom, the Association for Improvements in the Maternity Services (AIMS) was established in 1960 largely to campaign for women's rights to obtain a hospital delivery (at a time when demand for hospital beds exceeded supply). AIMS has since moved on to defending women's rights to give birth at home. The home birth campaign in Great Britain is now shared with another user organization set up with this as its specific platform—the Society to Support Home Confinements (SSHC), which was formed in 1974.

The first organizations of this type were set up in the late 1950s and early 1960s in the United Kingdom and the United States, but the main period of growth over most of Europe began in the mid-1970s. The AIMS *Directory of Maternity and Postnatal Care Organizations,* published in 1984, lists 135 organizations, many of them founded since 1980. Although some of these sound somewhat esoteric—for example, the National Association of Ovulation Method Instructors—many have well-known names. These include the Maternity Alliance, a network of interest groups that came together in 1980, and the Active Birth Movement, set up in 1982, in the aftermath of a protest against the ruling of one London obstetrician that all women delivering in his hospital would do so on their backs.

Figure 35 shows the motif of the *Active Birth Movement,* an early Greek relief showing a mother in a supported squatting position with the midwife waiting to catch the baby in front of her.

One outstanding example of cross-cultural continuity is the importance of personal experience as the starting point for these alternative activities. AIMS, for instance, began with the experiences of one woman who wrote to the press

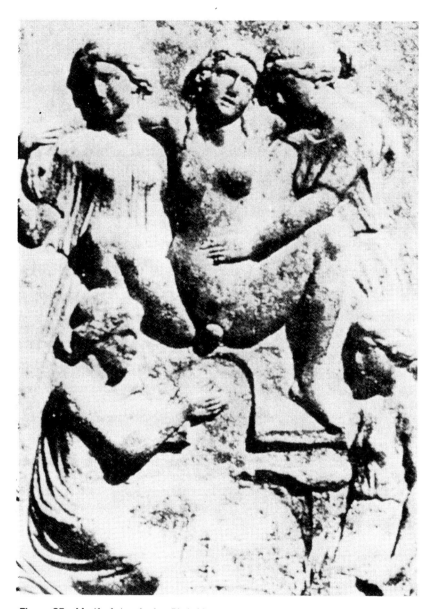

Figure 35 Motif of the *Active Birth Movement*.

about the appalling circumstances of her antenatal hospital stay (the original title of the organization was The Society for the Prevention of Cruelty to Pregnant Women). A Scandinavian home birth association was begun by a woman who wanted a home birth, but some women who were attracted to the organization were concerned mainly with improving hospital conditions; they subsequently split off from the parent organization to form a separate group, which has since become a large organization in its own right.

What are the functions of these user organizations? They include:

- Acting as a general information/resource center on birth issues (eight countries)
- Producing pamphlets and other informational material on rights/choices in childbirth and/or regular newsletters (eight countries)
- Serving as a forum for the exchange of news between parents and professionals (eight countries)
- Collecting information about the attitudes and services of individual care providers in the locality (four countries)
- Researching the attitudes and experiences of childbearing couples (seven countries)
- Providing a birth counseling service to help parents decide what kind of birth they want and how to get it (four countries)
- Helping to prepare couples for childbirth and parenthood through formal classes or informal discussions, using the experiences of parents rather than professional educators (five countries)
- Giving practical help with the formal complaints procedure in cases in which service users are dissatisfied with the treatment they have received (three countries)
- Raising funds for their own support or for health care resources directly (four countries)
- Organizing seminars and conferences (six countries)
- Representing the interests of childbearing couples to the media and to local and central government health departments (five countries)
- Organizing to deal with specific local/national issues, such as maternity hospital visiting hours and official harassment of home delivering couples or midwives (seven countries)

Which of these many activities predominates in any organization is determined by local circumstances and needs. For instance, the right to analgesia in childbirth has been a focal issue for user groups in Finland; a law was eventually passed securing this right. There is now concern among service users that the same law is being used by some care providers in the wrong way—namely, to persuade women to have analgesia when they do not really want it.

The oldest tradition in this field is undoubtedly educational preparation for parenthood. This had been the major concern of the National Childbirth Trust in the United Kingdom and the International Childbirth Education Association in

North America. Their work, stressing the importance of physical and psychological preparation for childbirth, is a direct response to the failure of the official services to see this as important. Whether by means of information or by using methods such as psychoprophylaxis and yoga, preparation for childbirth is not an integral part of the official mode of care provision, although it is one in which midwives frequently engage. It has thus been an obvious candidate for "semiprofessionalization" within user groups.

As well as the large national organizations, the alternative perinatal service field is dotted with a galaxy of smaller groups. Many of these are special interest groups; their focus may be Caesarean section, twin motherhood, premature delivery, miscarriage, breastfeeding, postnatal depression, or other issues. They exist to promote the sharing of information among people experiencing these events and to provide mutual support through crises.

ALTERNATIVE VERSUS OFFICIAL SERVICES

We use the term *alternative* to indicate some sort of basic opposition to the official services providing perinatal care. Illegal lay midwifery in the United States is perhaps the prototypical case. As this example suggests, alternative services are often not new; many mark a return to traditional forms of midwifery care. Ambulation in labor, vertical delivery, delayed cutting of the umbilical cord, and close mother-neonate contact in the early postpartum weeks—all of which feature in the alternative domain—are some examples of practices described by anthropologists studying nonindustrialized cultures. Lay midwives in Europe and North America today may use traditional herbal remedies and homeopathic cures or incorporate other ancient techniques, such as acupuncture, into the care they give to childbearing women. Sunshine as a treatment for neonatal jaundice has been uncovered as part of lay health care knowledge among the older generation in Scandinavia. Is phototherapy as used in modern neonatal intensive care units merely a case of rediscovering the wheel?

Within this alternative model of care, the diet of childbearing women has increasingly been singled out for attention. Whereas the official system may pay lip service to the importance of diet, within the alternative model it is regarded as an integral part of good prenatal care. In addition, alternative midwives may prescribe certain foods for specific complaints, such as celery for edema.

Given the historical and cross-cultural perspective outlined in Chapters 2 and 4, it seems more sensible to view the modern medicalization of perinatal care as an alternative to older traditional forms. Yet what is considered alternative is always a response to the dominant ideology. The dominant ideology in the industrialized world today is one of professional care.

Because of the association between alternative and traditional practices, many developing countries still heavily dependent on lay midwifery care do not yet have new, alternative services. The concerns of women in these countries lie more with the reproductive consequences of poverty and undernutrition and the scarcity of emergency medical resources, such as blood transfusion, than with concepts such as choice and postnatal mother-infant bonding. More than half of the world's births are unattended by trained personnel of any kind. Death rates of women in childbirth are commonly 200 times as great in developing countries as in the industrialized world; some 99 percent of the half-million maternal deaths each year occurs in these countries. The geographical differences in maternal deaths are the greatest in all public health statistics—a "neglected tragedy" in the words of Dr. Halfdan Mahler, former Director General of the World Health Organization. He believes this tragedy is "neglected because those who suffer it are neglected people, with the least power and influence over how national resources shall be spent." In this sense, traditional perinatal care is no golden age to which the alternative perinatal care movement either does or should envisage a return.

The definition of an alternative service depends to some extent on the circumstances of the individual country. For example, the location of labor and delivery in the same hospital room (rather than transferring women when the second stage of labor starts) constitutes an alternative practice in some countries. In those countries, the official system has conventionally insisted on a separation between labor and delivery care. In other countries, which lack an official tradition of moving a laboring woman into another room for delivery, women have not needed to demand change in this respect.

The financing of health care includes both government tax-based and public or private insurance-based systems. In all ten countries in our survey, antenatal, delivery, and postnatal care are available to the childbearing woman without the need for her to pay directly for these services at the time of use. The organization of perinatal care, however, differed between the countries in the survey. In three of the countries, perinatal care is provided almost wholly in institutions; general practitioners–obstetricians and midwives in independent practice do not exist. In the other seven countries, a woman may obtain care either at an institution (maternity hospital, clinic, or center) or through a doctor or midwife of her choice. Yet despite these variations, the modal pattern of perinatal care is the one described in Chapter 4: a hospital delivery preceded by antenatal care in a hospital clinic, often combined with some antenatal care provided in a non-hospital setting. Postpartum care is obtained in the hospital initially and later in the community. This is the official context into which alternatives are introduced. We found the following alternatives in at least some settings in the countries we visited:

- Attempts to provide continuity of care between antenatal and delivery personnel (eight countries)
- Birth rooms in hospitals furnished to have a home-like appearance (six countries)
- Flexibility with respect to delivery position (eight countries)
- Birth-chairs or birth-stools (six countries)
- A permissive attitude to the presence of relatives and friends at delivery (eight countries)
- No routine preparation (enema, bath, shave) for labor (seven countries)
- Acceptance of written delivery plans outlining a mother's wishes for the management of her delivery (five countries)
- No routine obstetrical interventions (e.g., episiotomy) (eight countries)
- The objective of a low intervention rate in general (e.g., induction or acceleration of labor, instrumental delivery, Caesarean section, intrapartum electronic fetal heart rate monitoring) (seven countries)
- Leboyer-style deliveries, involving dimming the lights at delivery and gentle treatment of the newborn (eight countries)

The existence of one alternative does not guarantee the existence of others. For example, in one country (with an insurance-financed health care system), the university hospitals are said to be open to alternative delivery positions and to have instituted a practice whereby the same team of midwives is responsible for giving antenatal and delivery care to each woman. At the same time, babies delivered by Caesarean section in one of these hospitals are routinely sent to special care for at least the first twenty-four hours of life. The reason for this is said to be to boost the pediatrician's fee.

A practice may also be more or less alternative. Frederick Leboyer's *Pour une Naissance sans Violence* advocated delayed cutting of the umbilical cord, bathing the newborn in water at body temperature instead of whisking it away to be weighed and examined, and keeping it close to its mother. A number of hospitals claiming to offer the option of a Leboyer delivery in fact preserve only some elements of the Leboyer formula, cutting the cord within minutes of delivery, weighing the baby, and omitting the bath routine (some frankly re-name this practice "modified Leboyer"). (See Figure 36.)

The capacity of alternative care options set up within the official hospital-based system genuinely to expand women's choice is limited in a number of ways. As we have already seen in the case of the midwife's work, hospitals are institutions that are bureaucratically administered and organized, with relatively inflexible rules and routines. It is difficult for hospital staff to be properly responsive to individual women's needs. The presence (even behind curtains) of modern obstetric technology may constitute a temptation to use it. Surveying *Home Away from Home: The Alternative Birth Center,* Linnea Klee gave this description in 1986:

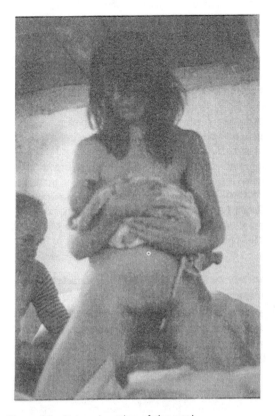

Figure 36 Delayed cutting of the cord.

Labor and delivery take place in a room furnished to resemble a bedroom. Often queen-size beds without stirrups or restraints are provided, although some alternative birth centres (ABCs) contain regular hospital beds covered with attractive bedspreads. The rooms may have carpeting, drapes, rocking-chairs, hanging plants, pictures on the wall. Equipment that is regarded as necessary by the obstetrical staff is usually hidden behind screens, in cupboards or drawers. . . .

Most importantly, each hospital draws up its own list of indications for non-eligibility for the ABC or for transfer out of the ABC to conventional labor and delivery rooms.

One implication of this is seen in our survey finding that alternative services that are provided in the hospital setting tend to be marked by higher intervention rates than those that operate entirely outside this context.

If the institution has an effect, so does experience. In a pilot project on midwifery practice in 500 planned home births in Britain, Marianne Scruggs has shown how increased experience affects perineal management. Over a four-year period, the episiotomy rate fell by 16 percent. There was an increase in the tear rate and also in the sutured tear rate, but the group with no sutures also increased considerably over this period.

The idea behind setting up alternatives—that the user should choose—has another important limitation put on it in practice. In all the countries we surveyed, as Klee reports for the alternative birth center (ABC) scene in the United States, those who provide alternative services mimic the practices of their official colleagues by some notion of risk to select women for alternative care. On the whole, only women considered obstetrically low-risk are seen as appropriate clients; women's own views about whether risk labels should be attached to them are generally not taken into account. An exception to this rule is a hospital in North America that has established a program of midwife care for high-risk women, with excellent results in terms of conventional mortality and morbidity outcome measures (see Chapter 6 for a more detailed discussion of this important question of who is at risk).

Place of Delivery

As we saw in Chapter 4, the trend over the past fifty years in many parts of Europe and North America has been toward increased rates of hospital confinement. In nine of the ten countries in our survey, however, at least some home births were reported to occur; figures ranged from less than 1 percent of all births to around 30 percent (See Figure 37.) Because the statistics do not distinguish between planned and unplanned home delivery, it is impossible to tell

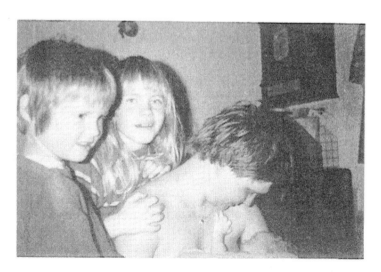

Figure 37 A family affair, born at home.

how many of these home births occur because the mother has chosen to give birth at home. One 1976 study in Norway (0.3 percent out-of-hospital deliveries, on a par with Denmark, Sweden, and the United Kingdom) found that one sixth of home births were planned.

In none of the ten study countries is home delivery technically illegal. In Denmark, national law permits home delivery, and a system has been set up within the midwife centers to meet the need for home births. Delivering a baby without attempting to secure the aid of a professionally qualified person is against the law in Sweden and the United Kingdom. In North America, nonattended home delivery is not illegal, but in some states the legal and professional medical pressure (which exists in many countries) against home delivery is sufficient to persuade some home birthers that concealment is the wisest course of action. In at least one of the countries we visited, there was evidence that some home births every year are not declared by the parents, despite the fact that this means loss of governmental child benefits.

Home delivery is a good example of the way in which the practical meaning of the concept of an alternative service varies from one country to another. Where the proportion of all babies delivered at home is only 1–2 percent, planned home deliveries are likely to be a symptom of the demand for alternative care. On the other hand, when the proportion is a third or more, home delivery is still normal or an accepted part of official perinatal care provision. Women do not have to engage in prolonged and often distressing arguments with service providers to secure the right to a home birth.

Advising women how best to succeed at this process has become a service offered by user organizations. The technique of verbal disarmament can be taught, as in the following examples based on real-life encounters between pregnant women and doctors:

Obstetrician: I find your wish for a home birth selfish and irresponsible. You're just looking for a fulfilling experience for yourself and not thinking about your baby.

Woman: I find your remarks deeply distressing. (*Pause.*) Have you ever considered that separating the interests of the unborn baby from the interests of the woman who is carrying it prepares the way for a totalitarian state?

Obstetrician: (Same remark.)

Woman: I find your remarks insulting to me as a person. (*Pause.*) Don't you think there's something wrong with a society which allows a man to say such things to a pregnant woman?

Obstetrician: (Same remark.)

Woman: I can see that my request threatens you in some way. (*Pause.*) In my case I would consider myself irresponsible if I handed over responsibility to you.

Obstetrician: (Same remark.)

Woman: I haven't come here to canvass your opinion, doctor. (*Pause.*) You don't know me well enough to question my motivation in this way.

Obstetrician: (Same remark.)

> *Woman:* I'm really sorry you find it necessary to say such things, doctor. (*Pause.*) I want you to know that it will damage our relationship.

These techniques are said to be very effective. They are certainly *not* the norm in doctor-patient encounters.

As we saw earlier, an important factor influencing the type of care provided is the type and financing of the health care system. Insurance-based health care systems may exhibit a bias toward one or another place of delivery (and type of antenatal care) by making one more expensive than another. In the Netherlands, for example, the State Insurance Fund will cover the cost of a hospital delivery and specialist care only for a pregnant woman who is certified as having an appropriate medical indication. Otherwise, the cost of hospital specialist care must be borne by the woman herself. One result of this situation is a demand for beds in university hospitals, which provide free care, among women who want a hospital delivery irrespective of their medical condition. Another is the rise in the incidence of certified medical conditions in pregnancy.

This situation in the Netherlands is a good illustration of the importance and complexity of the question of choice. There are reported to be some areas within the country with hospital delivery rates of around 90 percent, which are generating waves of protest from the local community, and other areas, also with high hospital confinement rates, where these are said to be what women want—for instance, because many of the men are on shift work and the women do not want to have their babies at home, unsupported by their partners. The women's choice in this case is a small maternity home that combines the social advantages of an institutional confinement with a respect for the delivery wishes of the individual women. On the whole, smaller maternity units seem more likely to do this.

France provides an illustration of almost an opposite case. In France, hospital delivery is a normal entitlement under the state health insurance scheme, whereas a home delivery with a midwife is not and must be paid for privately. The system of prenatal maternity allowances also weights the balance in favor of the official pattern of care, since these allowances cannot be claimed by the pregnant woman until she had undergone three medical examinations beginning before the end of the third month of pregnancy.

Making Money Out of Alternative Care

Alternative perinatal care has become big business in many countries. This may be partly because the size and bureaucracy of state-organized health care make the system unresponsive to innovation and change. The clearest example of this is probably the United States, where public hospitals have been quite resistant to the challenge of the alternative perinatal care movement, while a very wide range of alternative organizations has sprung up in the arena of private health care. A unique development in the United States has been the cooperative effort of providers and users in establishing alternative birth settings. The Childbearing Center in New York, one of the first such alternative institutions, was set up in 1975 as a cost-effective alternative to hospital birth that would hope to dissuade parents from home birth by providing them with its benefits without its supposed hazards.

When properly costed, alternative perinatal services are frequently cheaper than their official counterparts, in part—and paradoxically—because they rely on low-technology midwife-centered care. In the New York Childbearing Center, for instance, antenatal care is provided almost wholly by midwives, with two examinations by an obstetrician; its costs work out at about one third to one quarter of private hospital rates.

There are some eighty or ninety such centers in the United States, where pregnancies and births are managed by nurse-midwives with varying degrees of obstetrician back-up. Birth centers of this type also exist in Canada. All birth centers select clients according to their own predetermined risk criteria. Transfer rates to hospitals may be as high as 25 percent. The costs of birth center care commonly lie between those of conventional hospital care and care given by independent lay midwives. The term *birth center,* as used in Europe, may also describe an information/counseling/support center, which does not provide any facilities for birth at all.

The argument that midwife-provided care is cheaper clearly has its dangerous side, for a crucial element in the midwife's dilemma today is the link between her low professional status and its economic undervaluation. Money may be critical for those who provide alternative services. Partly for this reason, the major developments in the domain of alternative perinatal services are occurring in the private health care sector in seven of the ten countries we included in our study. One example is the provision by a private obstetrician of a delivery flat where women stay before, during, and after delivery with their families and/or friends. The obstetrician does the delivery, and the cost is refunded by the insurance system. He operates a strict risk system—no twins or breeches, for example—and has a 32 percent episiotomy and 96 percent suturing rate. The state insurance system makes an extra payment to the doctor for suturing even "one little stitch." A second example is a private maternity hospital, owed by a religious organization, which had very few clients until the organization hired a dynamic young obstetrician who quickly filled the hospital with patients, following the rule that the patient should have what she wants. Women are allowed to choose whether they have medication for delivery; the epidural rate is 37 percent.

In 1984, the costs of some commercially available alternative birthing equipment ran into thousands of dollars (Table 21). The most alternative of alternative services—lay midwives—may also charge a fee, as Margaret Reid, who studied lay midwives in North America, commented: "In the early days,

Table 21   Some Commercially Available Birthing Equipment

Product name (source)	Approximate current cost (US $)
Adel Bed (Adel Medical Limited, Portland, Oregon)	6800
Borning Bed (Borning Corporation, Spokane, Washington)	7940
Borning Genesis (Borning Corporation)	6500
Century Birth-EZ Chair (Century Manufacturing Company, Aurora, Nebraska)	6995
Stryker Bed (Stryker Corporation, Kalamazoo, Michigan)	5657

Source: McKay, 1984, p. 113.

lay midwives asked for little or no payment in return for services. Now, most midwives charge a fee ranging from $200 to $1500. True to their roots, though, many lay midwives would still do a birth for nothing, although food, wood, or other services remain an acceptable form of exchange."

Midwives and Alternative Perinatal Care

As the preceding examples show, alternative care is not always midwife-centered care. Yet midwives are key figures in the most alternative of alternative perinatal services: lay care. In some countries, midwives practice on the borders of legality, as members of underground networks that, in their ideologies and practices, constitute a direct challenge to the official system.

In the areas of North America where midwifery is illegal, there is obviously no official provision for midwifery training. In other areas where midwifery is permitted, the educational or training requirements are quite stringent. In Georgia, for example, midwives must be between twenty-one and sixty years of age, are obliged to register with the local health department, and must attend classes of instruction.

We have already seen how crucial is the distinction between midwife training based on nursing or separated from it. Many of those involved in alternative perinatal services see direct-entry midwifery as inherently preferable to a combined background of nursing and midwifery. The midwife who enters her profession without a nursing background is considered more likely to view pregnant women as people rather than as patients and to regard childbearing as a social instead of narrowly medical phenomenon. Direct-entry systems are thought more likely to encourage older women with personal experience of childbirth to enter midwifery, which is seen as important.

The following account of one woman's path to becoming a midwife illustrates an alternative method of training that we found in five of the countries we surveyed:

> I became a midwife after a bad experience of hospital delivery. When I got pregnant the next time, I started reading and thinking about a home birth. My midwife had to leave town, and then I decided to have the baby with a friend of mine who had had her two children at home and had seen three other births at home.
>
> After that, other women began asking me to their deliveries—just because I'd had a baby at home myself. I went to ten deliveries, all perfectly normal, and I asked my midwife if I could be her apprentice. There were two other women also wanting to be midwives, so there was a small group of us. We met once a week. We learned a lot from one another.

This lay midwife went on to start a prenatal clinic and birth counseling with her colleagues. They decided to work in pairs, so there would always be two of them at a delivery.

There are two distinct groups of lay midwives within the alternative service sector: young women who, like the midwife above, come to midwifery through negative personal experience of the official system, and older women in ethnic minority communities (gypsies, North American Indians, and so on) who act as granny midwives within their own subcultures. The younger women, if they are in touch with their traditional counterparts, familiarize themselves with the older methods and remedies, such as herbal medicine, and incorporate them into their practice. A good example of this historical link is, once again, The Farm in Tennessee. The Farm publishes birth and morbidity and mortality data showing the safety and effectiveness of the form of care they provide (within what is obviously to some extent an atypical population): a perinatal mortality rate of 8 per 1000 births, for example.

Lay midwives may work either with or without doctor back-up. In at least one country, doctors are liable to be fined if they are known to have helped a midwife with a home delivery, and in another a doctor known for his support of midwifery was threatened by his colleagues with total exclusion from hospital obstetrics. These are two among many sanctions applied by the official system to users and providers of alternative forms of care. One way of avoiding such confrontation is a pattern that is becoming increasingly popular in one of the ten countries: a lay midwife attends a woman in pregnancy, stays with her at home for the first stage of labor, then goes to the hospital with her as a support person; either she or a doctor will handle the actual delivery. In most places, it appears that enough individual obstetricians or general practitioners are sympathetic to the need for alternative care to allow some method of underground collaboration to be worked out with the lay midwives. Where this happens, the official services are performing the unusual function of a back-up to the alternative ones.

The following characteristics of lay midwives' work are common in all the countries where lay midwifery has emerged as an important alternative:

- Antenatal care based on a holistic approach to childbirth preparation, including counseling, dietary advice, massage, and yoga.
-· Emphasis on a good personal relationship between mother and midwife as essential (if the "vibrations" are bad, the midwife may refuse to take on the woman)
- Skeptical attitude toward routine obstetrical interventions
- Flexible attitude toward alternative birth positions, which means in practice that birth in an upright position is more likely to occur because the mother has been moving around freely in labor and has given birth in the most comfortable position for her, rather than because the midwife has insisted on upright delivery
- Low-cost compared with the official or other private services, with, in some countries, poor clients paying their lay midwives in kind

The role midwives play in alternative care reflects their role in the official system. On the whole, the weaker the position of midwives in the official services, the more pronounced their role in the alternative sector. Even in European countries with a comparatively strong tradition of midwifery as an autonomous profession, the midwives within or attached to hospital obstetrics tend to become doctors' assistants and/or to be replaced by nurses. The lead roles of the alternative perinatal service movement are played not by midwives but by doctors, and male doctors at that.

Two main lessons can be learned from the role of midwives in alternative care. One concerns the place of the law in regulating what midwives do. In general, in the countries we visited, midwives working within the hospital-based official system perform a range of activities and undertake a degree of responsibility that is much smaller than that legally allowed; working outside the system, however, their responsibilities and activities often exceed the legally permissible limit. The second lesson is thus that the most effective challenge to the male hegemony of the modern technological medical world may well lie in the domain of independent domiciliary practice.

Providing Alternative Perinatal Care

Challenges to the official perinatal services may emerge on an individual or collective basis. Individuals who begin working alone may join with one another. Being a revolutionary, even in a minor way, is a lonely business, and there is strength in numbers. In all countries with developed alternative services, their providers have organized themselves into local support groups. The example in the previous section of the midwife who chose her profession as a result of a bad experience with the official system is fairly typical of the way this comes about. The local support groups may make up underground networks of midwives willing to do home deliveries or of midwives in illegal practice who cannot afford to make public their activities. The point at which a local support group becomes a formal organization is sometimes hard to determine. If a formal organization is defined in terms of a name, a program of activities, formal membership criteria, and publications, five of the ten countries in our survey have formally constituted organizations for providers of alternative perinatal services.

In three countries, there are organizations whose membership is restricted to service providers, for example, a number of organizations of midwives and lay midwives in Canada and the United States. In the United Kingdom, the Association of Radical Midwives was founded in 1976. Disillusioned student midwives met to offer each other support during training and discovered a need for continuing mutual support and encouragement. Their choice of a title intentionally produced the acronym ARM, which also stands for the artificial rupture of membranes, a medical procedure they believed to be overused. The term *radical* was intended to refer to the "roots and origins of midwifery." The overall aim of ARM was "to restore the role of the midwife for the benefit of the childbearing woman and her baby." More specifically, its objectives were:

- To reestablish the confidence of the midwife in her own skills
- To share ideas, skills, and information
- To encourage midwives in their support of a woman's active participation in childbirth
- To reaffirm the need for midwives to provide continuity of care
- To explore alternative patterns of care
- To encourage evaluation of developments in the field

An analysis of the social backgrounds of ARM members showed that they were better educated than midwives in general and also significantly more likely to be direct entrants to the profession. A decade on, ARM remains an active and vociferous group within—or, rather, outside—the midwifery establishment. In 1986, a new organization, the Midwives' Information and Resource Service (MIDIRS), began an independent existence devoted to promoting midwifery education in a broad sense.

In the remaining two of the five countries with organizations of alternative service providers, membership is shared with the families who make use of these services. However, the provider constituency is the dominant element. The largest such organization, the National Association of Parents and Professionals for Safe Alternatives in Childbirth (NAPSAC), was formed in 1975. It has branches all over North America; affiliation can be on either an individual or a group basis. NAPSAC produces books, pamphlets, and a quarterly news-letter; it arranges conferences and seminars and maintains a directory of alter-native birth services.

In a sixth country, some providers of alternative care belong to what is predominantly a user group. Midwives outnumber doctors as members of these groups, although doctors are often overrepresented among the leaders. One organization, the Alternative Birth Crisis Coalition (ABCC) in the United States, was set up specifically to protect both providers and users of alternative care against official harassment.

Alternative Perinatal Services
and the Situation of Women

Many women active in the field of alternative perinatal care call themselves feminists, and some alternative perinatal service activities are regarded as form-ing an intrinsic part of the women's health movement.

The French organization, Femmes–Sages–Femmes (Women-Midwives), can be singled out as a unique merger of the alternative perinatal service move-ment and feminist politics. Originating in the mid-1970s as a midwife collec-tive, Women-Midwives grew into an organization of more than 1000 members, with the joint aim of improving the birthing conditions for mothers and the working conditions for midwives. To this end, representatives of the Ministry of Health and the government departments responsible for family welfare and for women's rights were invited to all their formal meetings.

Aside from the question of its association with organized feminism, the alternative perinatal service movement has other relationships with the position of women. As the eighteen-point program of the Parents and Childbirth group showed, the entitlement of mothers to financial benefits and to protection from discrimination in the employment field is often part of the agenda of user groups. Over much of the world, including Europe, the prevailing pattern of maternity benefits and employment protection legislation subjects many moth-ers to curtailed rights and choices and to a drop in their standard of living, which is hardly conducive to the goal of maternal and child welfare.

The direct and indirect effects of employment on pregnancy and its out-come have the status of a public issue in some places; there is a growing emphasis in some countries on the reproductive hazards of some branches of women's work, for example, in chemical factories. By comparison, very little attention has been directed to the reproductive hazards of women's unpaid work in the home. State-provided or state-subsidized domestic help in the perinatal period exists in only three of the ten countries and is an issue taken up by some user groups. The one European country, the Netherlands, that is the envy of all the others in this respect has an extensive, highly organized system of trained maternity aides, financed under the State Health Insurance scheme. Maternity aides provide mothers with up to eight hours of help per day for seven to ten days following childbirth. An interesting conflict is developing here between the maternity aide system and alternative forms of care. Progressive midwives are finding that the traditional official training of the aides does not easily lend itself to new midwifery ideas and techniques.

THE OFFICIAL SYSTEM RESPONDS

Has this tide of alternative activity had any impact on the official system? One mode of response is incorporation: flowery wallpaper in hospital delivery rooms, modern delivery beds masquerading as nineteenth-century antiques, and encouragement to childbearing women to develop their own birth plans. There are also more subtle moves afoot, such as the new interest among obstetricians in fetal movement counting as a perinatal monitoring strategy. Although fetal movement counting is based on the idea that mothers have some sense of their fetuses' health, it asks mothers to talk the quantitative language of obstetricians rather than encouraging obstetricians to listen to mothers' own qualitative accounts of fetal health.

Incorporation may be symptomatic of a benign attitude on the part of the perinatal health care establishment to the challenge of the alternative movement. However, there are also other responses. Particular debates fueled by the arguments of user organizations, such as the debate about induction of labor, have had an effect on official perinatal practice, although it is extremely difficult to disentangle these effects from other concurrent changes, such as an increased critical awareness among obstetricians themselves of some of the hazards of modern childbirth practices.

Another reaction is considerably less benign and consists of a range of sanctions applied to those who use and provide alternative forms of care. Some examples are:

- Official efforts to pass new legislation controlling maternity care practices (two countries)
- Prosecution (threatened or actual) of lay midwives or trained midwives practicing without doctor back-up (four countries)
- Prosecution of couples delivering at home without a "professional attendant" (one country)
- "Legal abandonment" by doctors of women requesting home delivery (three countries)
- Threatened loss of employment/security for doctors who actively support home delivery/lay midwifery (three countries)
- Exclusion of home-delivery midwives and their clients from hospitals (when conditions requiring hospital transfer develop) (four countries)

CONTINUITIES AND CONTRADICTIONS
WITHIN THE ALTERNATIVE MOVEMENT

Women's protest against the lack of information, choice, and power available to them within the official, medically dominated perinatal health services reflects the disablement of the individual within the modern professionalized and bureaucratized state. It also signals the continuing oppression of women as a group and is a reaction against the decline in midwife-managed childbirth, which is one main theme of this book. The pattern of protest is varied and difficult to document, but, to sum up, it could be said that the alternative perinatal service movement has the following characteristics:

1 *It is international.* Despite the differences between nations in health care systems, health care needs, and so on, users and providers of alternative perinatal services share a sense of participation in a worldwide movement, with a core of common aims and strategies. For example, English midwives migrate to run a midwifery association in North America, and midwives and seekers of home birth within Scandinavia exhibit a profound disregard for the usual national frontiers. Cross-fertilization of ideas is common. A highly efficient underground information network makes it possible for childbearing women with sufficient motivation (and money) to find the type of care they desire—if not in their own country then in another. This international flavor of alternative care was demonstrated by the holding of the first International Conference on Active Birth in London in October 1982.

2 *It is commercial.* In several countries, alternative perinatal services are fast becoming an attractive commercial proposition. While it is perhaps inevitable that the private sector should experience the fastest and most untrammeled growth of alternative options, this does not necessarily further the choice, freedom, and control of the mass of childbearing women, whose care will always, for financial reasons, be confined to the public health care sector.

3 *It is inclined to its own orthodoxies.* Radical political and social movements that arise in response to one set of orthodoxies are in turn liable to generate their own. There is more than a hint within the alternative perinatal service movement of precisely that attitude of inflexibility to which the movement was a response. For instance, being forced to walk around in labor or deliver one's baby standing up is as much a limitation of freedom as being forced to lie still and deliver in a supine position.

4 *It is organized around the concept of childbearing as a normal, social process.* The alternative perinatal movement is not simply a repository of herbal remedies and enthusiastic home deliveries. At its center stands an alternative model of perinatal care provision. Essential to this alternative model is a move away from the medical paradigm of childbearing, with its emphasis on clinically determined risk—the division of pregnant women into those for whom childbirth is somehow intrinsically risky and those for whom it is not expected to be so. Some people providing alternative care even take the view that those women most at risk according to conventional medical criteria are those who most need alternative forms of care. At the same time, to play safe, others who provide alternative care are operating their own definition of risk, which may be different from the prevailing official definitions but is, nevertheless, based on the same approach. An important element in this alternative model of perinatal care provision is a sharing of what is known, and what is not known, about the best way of obtaining health and survival for mothers and children. Decision-making should also be shared. This is an important principle, even if it is not always possible to follow it in practice.

5 *It represents an alliance between midwives and childbearing women.* Alternative perinatal services give great prominence to the role of the female midwife and to the way in which her autonomy as the manager of normal childbearing has been diluted over the years. Midwives and childbearing women often have an underlying coalition of interests in the way in which childbearing is managed now and in the future. The branches of the alternative movement in which mothers and midwives have recognized this underlying coalition and have organized together have been the most successful in securing change. Furthermore, although organized protest against obstetrician-controlled perinatal care is confined to industrialized countries, many of its lessons are applicable to the Third World. In Third World countries, 60–80 percent of all births are under the care of traditional birth attendants, and in many a laissez-faire attitude prevails toward these attendants: their practices are neither encouraged nor discouraged. Gradually, however, over the past ten years, it has come to be accepted that indigenous practitioners, such as traditional birth attendants, can function within modern Western health care systems. Up to 1982, traditional midwives had been given some degree of formal training and upgrading in forty-four countries. Most of these programs were local rather than national in character: only seventeen of the forty-four countries had incorporated traditional midwives at the national level into the health care system.

As far as human beings learn lessons from history, it would seem that at least two lessons need to be learned from the activities described in this chapter. First, the exclusion from childbirth of autonomous midwifery restricts the care options available to childbearing women and inevitably promotes the definition of childbearing as a pathological, medicalized process. Second, while the dominant myth of the age is that official medicine is scientific and effective, whereas lay alternatives to it are not, it is often the case that official medicine is neither effective nor scientific, while alternative forms of care may be both. In their attack on official medical services for not being sufficiently based on scientific principles, it is essential, however, that the providers and users of alternative care evaluate their own practices. It is, after all, the aim of all perinatal care—whether official, alternative, or traditional—to promote the safety, health, and happiness of mothers, children, and the community in general and to find the strategies, no matter their origins or practitioners, that maximize the achievement of these ends.

Chapter Six

Who Is at Risk?

The modern definition of childbearing as a dangerous experience that must be medically controlled has at its heart the idea of risk. Many aspects of life are risky, but we make no attempt to prevent people from exercising their democratic right to expose themselves to such risks if they so choose. In the area of childbirth, the development of modern obstetric practice means that women are not allowed to determine for themselves the risk they take in having a baby. At the present time in the industrialized world, the risk of a woman herself dying in childbirth is about 1 in 10,000 (live births and stillbirths); deaths of babies around the time of birth are around 10 per 1000. Table 22 shows the risk of dying run by individuals engaged in a number of everyday activities, which is roughly equivalent to the risk of dying in childbirth for a woman in a developed country today (to find equivalents for the risk to the baby, multiply the figures in Table 22 by a factor of ten).

For many years, obstetricians have been fascinated by the idea that it ought to be possible to predict which pregnant women will develop complications. Many different risk-scoring systems have been developed and tried, but all have been shown to have flaws: they fail to identify some women who do have

**Table 22   One in 10,000 Risk of
Death, from Different Causes**

75 cigarettes
5000 miles by car
25,000 miles by air
2-1/2 hours rock climbing
10 hours canoeing
33 hours being a man aged 60 years
100 days being a boy aged 12 years
100–200 weeks of typical factory work

Source: Nicholson, 1986.

problems and incorrectly point the finger at some who do not. Most such risk systems combine social and medical factors. One example is included in Appendix 2.

The definition of risk is thus central to the medical model of birth. What are the consequences of this for the way in which childbearing women are cared for by both doctors and midwives? Much of this chapter is based on material prepared by a group of Danish women[1] (two midwives, one obstetrician-to-be, one sociologist, and one psychologist) who formed themselves into a special interest group around the issue of home birth. After a time, they began to see that it was impossible to talk about home birth without confronting and disentangling the medical idea that childbirth is too risky for women themselves to have much say in it. In turning their attention to the ideology of risk and its implications for maternity care today, the group identified a number of critical elements in the idea of childbirth as an inherently risky event. In the sections that follow, which represent a translated and edited version of the document on risk produced by the group, each of these component ideas is itemized in turn, its content critically examined, and alternative strategies proposed. In the process, many of the key issues discussed in this book concerning the present and future of midwifery are subjected to intimate and revealing scrutiny.

PROBLEMS WITH THE RISK APPROACH

Item 1. The risk approach defines the birth situation as the most important issue within maternal health and maternity care, at the expense of many other decisive phases and circumstances from the beginning of the pregnancy to the end of the postpartum period.

---

[1]J. Moeller, S. Houd, U. Marcussen, D. Gannik, H. Wolf.

No culture exists in which birth is unimportant. All cultures rank pregnancy, birth, and the postpartum period somewhere between sublimity and illness, and this ranking is of importance for cultural myths, rituals, and expectations.

It is of great importance to parents in our culture that the baby they are expecting is born alive and viable, but the risk approach has exploited this wish. The goal of maternity care is to contribute to the birth of a healthy baby, while preserving the mother's life and health. However, in the risk approach, problems of perinatal mortality and morbidity have been given undue prominence. (See Figure 38.)

The goal of a low perinatal mortality rate has become a question of international prestige. Obstetricians worldwide concentrate on the goal of reducing the perinatal mortality rate in their country a little below that of neighboring countries. Because ours is a competitive society, such ranking in comparison to others can succeed economically: even when the rating is good or extremely good, more money may still be poured into high technology maternity care.

Birth has become important for a negative reason—the wish to avoid mortality (and morbidity) at any price. However, birth is important because it is a unique and central event in the whole physical, mental, social, and cultural life of the woman, the baby, and the family. It is important that as many babies as possible are brought into the world alive, but even when this does not happen birth is still an important event. A baby has not been successfully brought alive and well into the world until it has been integrated in the daily life of the family.

Among the issues that are not being taken seriously by the medical and

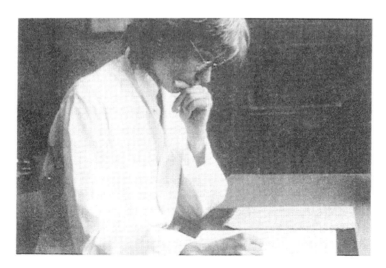

Figure 38 Looking for risk.

epidemiological experts are the mother's work environment before the pregnancy, women's double workload, the relationship between the parents, sexuality, women's emotional reactions when first feeling fetal movements, the influence of diet on health, economic and social conditions, mental preparation for becoming parents, attachment to the baby after the birth, and breastfeeding.

Item 2. Because the birth situation is defined as the most important issue in such restricted ways, the contribution of midwives, general practitioners, social workers, psychologists, health visitors, physiotherapists, relaxation teachers, and others in this area is weakened and devalued.

The division of pregnant and birthing women into risk groups has determined the referral system: at the top the obstetricians, next the general practitioners, then the midwives, and at the bottom all the others. Referral is mainly one way: into the consultant units for evaluation and possibly for birth. The referral of pregnant women from midwife to general practitioner takes place because of minor problems, and there are a few referrals from midwives and general practitioners to social workers and health visitors. It is unthinkable that an obstetrician on his or her own initiative should refer a pregnant woman to a midwife so that the midwife could evaluate whether it would be better to have a home birth for family-related or psychological reasons.

The rule of thumb of the risk approach is that the more risk factors one acknowledges, the more risks can be countered, and the fewer complications of pregnancy and birth should occur. This has an impact on many midwives and general practitioners, who become more concerned about finding something wrong with the pregnancy than finding anything right with it. The problems they find are to be taken care of not by themselves but by the specialists. Thus, many midwives and general practitioners learn to devalue their own expert clinical and psychosocial skills.

Item 3. The "patient" becomes a passive object.

That the "patient" is treated as an inanimate object is illustrated by, for example, a recently published information booklet in Danish for pregnant women, *Et barn skal foedes* (*A baby is to be born,* Munksgaard, 1983). Machines and interventions are shown, with the parts of the body of the woman, confined to her bed, on which the individual instruments are used. The healthy, normal birth has retreated—or been pushed—into the background.

Being deprived of responsibility is a relief to some people, while others may feel humiliated by it (Figure 39). Women in the latter category are often described as selfish and irresponsible, and obstetricians may be reluctant to listen to what they have to say. Communication in the system is not designed to elicit feedback and act on its consequences.

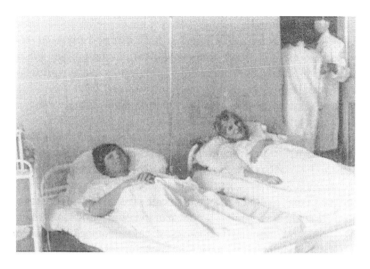

Figure 39 Passive patients.

Birth preparation classes are in theory places in which dissatisfaction with the role of the patient can be expressed. Generally speaking, however, this only happens in those few places where the courses are not attached to midwifery centers or hospitals. Otherwise, the main function of the classes is to give information rather than to encourage dialogue.

It is foreign to the nature of the risk approach to respect the birthing woman as a mature, independent sexual being engaging in an active, creative process.

Most pregnant women put up with the system, especially if their pregnancy has been placed in a risk group. The system ignores the stress that may be a consequence of exposing pregnant women to numerous tests. Tests often show small deviations from normal results, which are difficult to interpret and cause anxiety.

Item 4. Obstetricians consider themselves advocates for the unborn and the newborn baby.

Pleading the cause of the child is a positive thing, but it becomes something negative when the mother herself and the family as a whole are not considered.

Treating pregnant and birthing women as objects allows obstetricians to regard them as a kind of incubator in which one can put a baby or from which one can remove a baby according to what one feels will serve the baby best. Of course, obstetricians do not wish to interfere with the other main function of this incubator, which is, a few days after the birth, taking the major responsibility for the child's upbringing and welfare for the next sixteen to eighteen years.

Two situations particularly illustrate this mistrust of the mother as her child's best advocate: when it is suspected that the unborn baby is not getting enough nourishment and is therefore developing too slowly (growth retardation), and when the baby dies in connection with the birth.

In the first case, obstetricians use the term *concentration camp syndrome*. The uterus is regarded as a concentration camp, and obstetricians rescue the baby from it. According to one leading Danish obstetrician, this syndrome is the cause of approximately one third of all perinatal mortalities.

When the baby dies in connection with the birth, the death may often be felt as some kind of failure of the birth attendant. Psychological defenses, implied in the denial of the existence of death, break down. The birth attendant is confused and unable to support the woman in her grief or to take her feelings seriously. Instead, the mother is advised to have another baby as quickly as possible. Or she is supposedly cheered up by being reminded that she has other children at home.

Item 5. From being a demanding, but basically natural, event, birth in the risk approach is primarily regarded as a life-threatening situation.

Forty years ago, maternal mortality was approximately thirty times higher than now, and perinatal mortality was some ten times higher. Nobody wants to return to such conditions, but, given the present good results, one wonders why obstetricians still argue in favor of all women giving birth in a consultant unit rather than in a smaller ward, in a clinic, or at home.

Their main argument is that perinatal mortality has fallen as births in consultant units have risen; births in other places will be beset by unpredictable conditions leading to sudden transfer. Births in consultant units involve risks that are rarely or never mentioned by obstetricians.

Consultant units tend to be large. This increases risk, because several people, generally unknown to the mother, take over from each other in the management of individual births. There is the risk of overtreatment in a hierarchic system and the risk of infection—to mention only two of the most obvious hazards.

Even though perinatal mortality today is low and many births take place in consultant units, there is no guarantee that a further degree of specialization, with a possible fall in perinatal mortality, will benefit women with normal pregnancies and births. It is possible that perinatal mortality for normal pregnant women who give birth in consultant units is higher today than for similar women giving birth elsewhere. This would be concealed, however, in improved mortality figures for high risk groups.

So far as home birth is concerned, it is unfortunate that the statistics of many countries do not differentiate between planned home births and other births outside hospital, such as very fast unplanned births. Surveys from the Netherlands and the United Kingdom show a low perinatal mortality in planned home births.

The more successful the risk approach is in proclaiming birth a life-threatening situation, the more fear the general public has of what can happen at birth. Fear brings about less confidence in one's own abilities and creates negative expectations. The risk approach thus becomes a self-fulfilling prophecy.

Item 6. Birth is defined as a life-threatening situation requiring surveillance, control, and intervention at any sign of deviation from the "normal."

This issue raises questions about a whole series of technical procedures used during pregnancy and birth, including amniocentesis, hormone analysis, electronic fetal monitoring, ultrasound screening, induction of labor, Caesarean section, vacuum extraction and forceps, episiotomy, and use of drugs and anesthesia.

When amniocenteses are carried out mid-pregnancy, severe fetal malformations can be diagnosed in only some cases. There is also a problem in deciding who should have the tests. At least one obstetrician has suggested carrying out amniocenteses on all pregnant women—an act that would throw suspicion on, and medicalize, all pregnancies. The risk of diagnostic errors is rarely mentioned.

At the beginning of the pregnancy, hormone analyses are of importance in only a few cases. It now looks as if most obstetricians only attach importance to these results in certain risk cases, and then only as one among several examination parameters.

Electronic fetal monitoring (EFM) is an example of a technique that rapidly found a niche for itself. In 1976 the need for EFM was used as an argument for recommending the centralization of births. Many obstetricians today, however, would be of the opinion that EFM should not be used as a routine procedure.

One hears relatively little about the problem of interpreting correctly the results of EFM. Correct interpretation of this technology is necessary to avoid hasty and unnecessary intervention. The same caution applies to the risk of infection or other damage to the baby from the use of scalp electrodes. Finally, EFM can involve the use of ultrasound, but as yet it is not known whether continuous low dose ultrasound has a harmful effect.

Ultrasound screening is a great hit today. This method of fetal monitoring is often described as one of the greatest advances in modern obstetrics. It is understandable that people become excited over new developments and that people who speak against these may be ignored. Experiments with animals in the United States indicate chromosome mutations following ultrasound screening. Other problems, including next-generation effects, such as reduced fertility, are rarely referred to as possibilities.

As far as the risk approach leads to the recommendation of mass use of a technique, it is dangerous. A more responsible course of action would be to proceed slowly and carefully with a new technique, using it only when it is impossible to find other reasonable, thoroughly tested solutions. The routine introduction of ultrasound screening in obstetrics has had the same sort of negative influences as many other new techniques: midwives and doctors inevitably spend less time and energy using and extending their clinical experience. Perhaps the use of new techniques should be reserved for the old clinicians. Then, such techniques would be limited to support of clinical diagnoses, and new doctors would still be able to learn their trade.

Less technical and resource-demanding examinations and tests tend not to be valued as much as new techniques. For example, fetal movement counts involve only three technical aids: paper, a pencil, and a watch. Surveys have shown that fetal movement counts can help obstetricians in cases of genuine high-risk pregnancy not to overreact to falling hormone levels and dubious EFM results. This method also puts the mother at the center of the examination field. One reason why fetal movement counts have met with opposition in Denmark is because people have used this method to try to identify threatened intrauterine fetal death by ordering all pregnant women to perform fetal movement counts from the thirty-second week of pregnancy on. Some pregnant women enjoy surveying the activity of their fetuses in this way, but others experience increased anxiety: "It's not enough that you're nervous about what they'll say when you go for prenatal care, now they also ask you three times a week to sit at home in your living-room with your hand on your stomach and be frightened!"

Another, less technical test is symphysis-fundal height, which involves measuring with an ordinary tape measure from the top of the symphysis to the top of the uterus to register its growth. This test has been used in Sweden for more than ten years. This method has been evaluated in three obstetrical units in Denmark and been found to be useful; it also has the advantage of being cheap and harmless.

Induction of labor has been a key issue since the early 1970s. There are other, less technical types of induction apart from the use of artificial hormonal methods. These include advising pregnant women to engage in increased physical activity or sexual activity with orgasm, or to take castor oil or other laxatives. A popular medical method not included in the official statistics of maternity care is "stripping of the membranes." This is often accompanied by bleeding. No research has been done to find out about the potential effectiveness or hazards of this intervention.

The rates of Caesarean section, vacuum extraction, and forceps are very different in different countries. In most places over the past fifteen years, there has been a 50 percent increase in the rate of Caesarean section and an even higher increase in the use of vacuum extraction.

The risk of being delivered by Caesarean section in Denmark was one in twenty-five in 1970, and in 1980 it was one in nine. This increase is normally explained by reference to three factors. First, Caesarean section is recommended in breech presentations, especially in women having their first babies; this group of women is increasing in numbers as a proportion of all births. Second, EFM makes it easier to identify fetal anoxia and to intervene by doing a Caesarean section. Third, an increasing number of labors are marked by a lack of progress, making Caesarean section advisable.

Episiotomy is performed in just under 40 percent of all births in Denmark. It is generally not considered an intervention, probably because it is so routine as to be considered normal. There are two obstetrical arguments in favor of performing episiotomy: when the baby is estimated to weigh less than 2500 g and cannot stand too much pressure on its head, or when there is not enough room for the baby to get out without tearing the mother's perineum. Very little research has yet been done to investigate the validity of these arguments or the consequences of this intervention, for example, for mother-infant bonding or as long-term perineal pain and sexual or psychological difficulties. Similarly, little research has been carried out on the effectiveness, acceptability, and side effects of drugs, including anesthetics, given to women during labor and delivery.

In short, the risk approach model of birth as a life-threatening situation has led to increasing surveillance, control, and intervention.

Item 7. The risk approach is scientifically awkward. It is logically impossible to define the abnormal without first defining the normal, with all its possible variations. Obstetricians are particularly deficient in knowledge of variations in what is normal. Their answer is to define normality retrospectively: "No birth can be said to be normal until it is over" (Figure 40).

Biomedical science, in which the risk approach is embedded, borrowed its basic methods of measurement from the fields of physics and chemistry. In those fields, it is a question of laboratory studies of single elements and of statistical calculation methods: a question of a scientific view that presupposes that everything can be objectively measured, weighed, and evaluated and that assumes the existence of one and only one scientific truth.

Prenatal diagnosis of amniotic fluid is one example of a test carried out according to this paradigm. It is assumed that it will eventually be possible to define what is normal by carrying out a sufficiently large number of amniocenteses. This is, of course, an absurdity. This way one can only choose to say what one accepts as normal. The question is, who is to make the choice?

Today, in the field of prenatal diagnosis, there are often borderline cases where it is not clear that something is wrong, but, on the other hand, it cannot

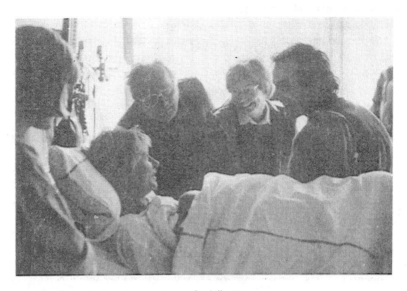

Figure 40   Normal after the event: a safe delivery.

definitely be said that the finding is normal. Who is to decide whether the pregnancy is to continue? The doctors can choose not to tell the parents about such findings, or they can let the parents make the choice of interrupting or continuing the pregnancy. They can also evaluate which parents would be capable of choosing for themselves and who would not. Often, they can choose to recommend to the parents interruption of the pregnancy.

Item 8. When the thesis of the risk approach—that no birth can be said to be normal before it is over—has succeeded in making most people uneasy, obstetricians offer to take responsibility for all pregnancies and births by centralizing care in highly specialized maternity units.

At some stage, a change has occurred in who is responsible for normal birth. Recommendations for maternity care in Denmark contain an interesting comment that may have worldwide relevance to the role of the midwife. It comes in Regulation No. 633 of the 1972 *Regulations Concerning the Organization of Midwifery in Denmark:*

> Although the midwives did a commendable job in caring for pregnant women during pregnancy, prophylaxis in the modern sense was out of the question for an isolated midwife, partly because she lacked the necessary examination apparatus and partly because the extent of the prophylaxis depended on the individual midwife's job possibilities and therefore could not become systematic and uniform.

It appears . . . that one of the reasons why the system does not any longer function satisfactorily has to do with the decentralized organization of maternity care. The board therefore thinks that an overall organization under one unified management should be aimed at. . . . As it is the hospitals which are, or will become, crucial for birth, the board has decided that maternity care as a whole should be a hospital responsibility. . . . The medical management of the entire maternity care system, both within and outside hospitals, should be transferred to the chief of the gynecological/obstetrical consultant unit in the county.

By instituting this central organization, it will be possible to cure the isolation of the individual midwife. At the same time, she can retain her position, not as *the* central but as *a* central person in the maternity care.

This conclusion was a decisive factor in removing maternity care from the midwife and transferring it to the obstetrician.

Item 9. In consultant units, obstetricians and pediatricians work to decrease the limits of the lives it is possible to save, and in so doing they stress the risk of being born and increase the demand for technological provision for very small sick babies and all other possible negative outcomes.

It is well known that close and warm contact between the newborn and the mother is important for the health of both (Figure 41). However, this knowledge is being allowed to languish. Many obstetricians and pediatricians working to save very ill babies do not see the advantages of close mother-baby contact for healthy babies.

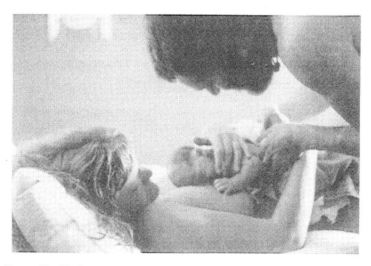

Figure 41   Mother and baby, with father, after the birth.

Obstetricians and pediatricians have achieved good results, but they have not succeeded in reducing the percentage of babies born with a weight below 2500 g.

Item 10. Survival is not the same thing as ideal care.

We have said that the risk approach may gradually assume the character of a self-fulfilling prophecy. The only way to stop this development is—in our opinion—to appreciate survival as a necessary, but not sufficient, condition for ideal care and then really start doing something about it. Survival loses its meaning if, at the same time, priority is not given to considering the issue of ideal care. Survival and ideal care are not synonymous, and ideal care does not automatically follow from survival.

Psychological research during the past fifteen years has rapidly expanded our knowledge of the potential capacities of the newborn. This knowledge also applies to the ill newborn. These infants get a difficult start in life and do not need to have their difficulties increased by being deprived of the necessary stimulation of the mother-infant couple's first union, skin to skin and face to face.

Even after uncomplicated births in modern consultant units, it is common for babies to be removed from their mothers for mucus extraction and to be generally checked over. If one inquires about the reason for this, the answer will be that it is the safest thing to do because even normal babies may have swallowed amniotic fluid. Where are the studies that form the background for this treatment? Treatment for the ill newborn is applied to the healthy newborn, just to be on the safe side. If a treatment seems to be effective on one type of patient, one has an obligation to "let everybody benefit from it." That healthy individuals may become ill or may lose by being suspected of being ill is an assumption foreign to the risk approach.

Because of the risk approach, more and more people are being subjected to more and more, increasingly expensive, treatment.

Item 11. To define birth as simultaneously most important and very dangerous is not a sign of comprehensive knowledge but rather of limited knowledge.

Maternity care based on the medical risk approach can and should be questioned. It is a manifestation of a modern mechanistic philosophy of life.

So far, the risk approach model has been strong enough to resist competition from other models. Recently, however, pressure from critical service users has caused some rethinking among providers of maternity care. Through fear of losing ground, they now seriously propose experiments with, for example, home birth in institutions.

If the good results that maternity care based on the risk approach has achieved during the past fifteen years are to be preserved, all doctors and midwives must stop considering maternity care their own internal problem. Providers of maternity care should ask users and other professionals, such as health visitors, psychologists, and social workers, to help them evaluate what they are doing well, what they are doing badly, and what should be changed. Medical knowledge, which is based on experience with ill people, must be complemented with knowledge based on women's own experiences and the knowledge of other professionals. It must also be complemented with knowledge derived from experiences with healthy pregnancy and birth processes.

The quality of maternity care is of interest to the whole of society. Birth statistics need to be extended to include ways of preventing problems other than the medical and economic. Research projects can take the questions and experience of the users as their starting point. How else, except by confinement, can pregnant women be relieved? Are the arguments in favor of episiotomy valid? What is the real value of the pudendal block and other forms of pain relief during birth? Can the fear of birth attendants influence the birth process? Are perinatal mortality and the mother's subjective feeling of security connected? Which different factors provoke birth depression? Do child abuse and maternity care have anything to do with each other?

The history of medicine is rich in examples of uncritical enthusiasm for new techniques. The history of medicine is also, unfortunately, just as rich in examples of opposition to simpler solutions. It took more than thirty years for Semmelweiss' ideas about the origins of puerperal fever to be accepted.

ALTERNATIVES TO THE RISK APPROACH

Item 12. In our pluralist industrial society, there is a need for health services to offer primary prevention throughout pregnancy, birth, and the postpartum period.

To give primary preventive health care, doctors must revise their traditional role as people who must be capable of instant diagnosis and immediate intervention. Pregnancy is not an illness that can be cured only if one does this or that. Pregnancy is a new condition, a preparatory phase, a time of maturing that ideally is lived in such a way that the child, when born, will have good parents (Figure 42).

The first task of midwives and doctors must be to discuss with the woman, and preferably also her partner, how the parents themselves look upon the situation and what possible problems they have or anticipate having. The couple must be told the kinds of support that are available to them and who can give

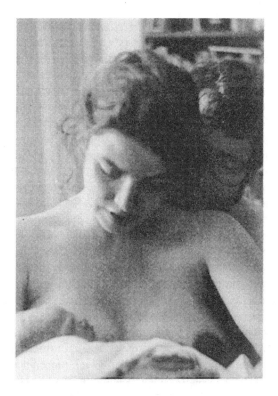

Figure 42   Child and parents.

these. The meaning of the concept of primary prevention in relation to pregnancy and birth is that it is essentially a question of strengthening the woman to give birth and take care of her own baby. The mother is the central person in maternity care, and the midwife, the doctor, and other health workers are her assistants (Figure 43).

Positive expectations are important. The woman's expectation of being capable of handling pregnancy, birth, and the postpartum period should be strengthened in such a way that she dares to believe in herself and her abilities. To manage a family with small children requires a firm foundation of physical and emotional strength, and the tasks of health workers should be extended to facilitate this.

Item 13. Primary prevention does not consist of surveillance and control, but of rendering support that is carefully adapted to the needs of the individual woman in her particular situation.

Surveillance and control inevitably lead to some loss of control for the person being surveyed. Although some pregnant and birthing women find it convenient to give up control in this way, midwives and doctors are not thereby exempted from their duty not to deprive any person of a desired responsibility.

The concept of primary support person or people is an important one. The objective of the primary support team should be to support the woman or couple in making appropriate choices and decisions about the type of care they wish to have.

Midwives or general practitioners can act as primary support people for childbearing women; so can other health workers, such as health visitors. The support task of health workers must also be seen in the context of the woman's existing social networks or relatives and friends.

Item 14. In order for the health services to render primary prevention, the following are required: (1) small hospital wards offering personal contact to women who spend time in them; (2) awareness on the part of the staff of their own limitations and resources, both professional and personal; and (3) close cross-disciplinary cooperation between health workers concerned with maternity care.

It is in society's interest to find an optimal model for providing maternal and child health services. Perinatal mortality and morbidity statistics have traditionally been used to evaluate the success of maternity services, but they provide limited data. It is important to consider measures of the quality of care.

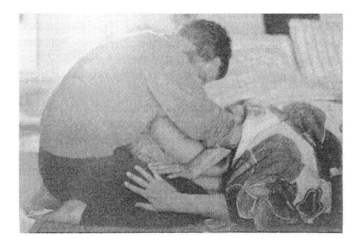

Figure 43 Support person.

Item 15. A model of maternity care based on primary prevention must use a comprehensive approach, both in its science and in its philosophy. It should use both qualitative and quantitative scientific methods to evaluate its effectiveness.

The terms *quantitative* and *qualitative* cannot be said to be adequate because quantitative research may well have important qualitative aspects, and vice versa. As yet, however, new terms have not been found.

One difference between quantitative and qualitative research methods is that quantitative methods tend to limit the number of investigated factors; on the other hand, they can work with a very large number of units (e.g., people), whereas qualitative research may include many factors but tends to be limited to a small number of units. The results of qualitative research are often very complex to present and interpret, while quantitative research can be expressed in figures that may look much simpler.

A further critical element in the comprehensive approach to providing and evaluating maternity care based on primary prevention is that underlying political ideologies very often exist and need to be articulated. All human attitudes, actions, and research are necessarily informed by political positions and values.

Item 16. The results of a system of maternity care based on primary prevention need not be less good than those produced by the risk approach system.

We find discussing maternity care extremely difficult. The difficulty lies in the fact that obstetricians tend to present their figures and arguments as if they had an absolutely objective validity. The problem derives from the fact that, although the risk approach has many negative consequences, it has provided good results in genuinely high risk cases, precisely because of the knowledge that has been accumulated about pathological pregnancy and birth processes. Objecting to the risk approach is also difficult because the idea of risk is a product of the culture in which we live. Because of this, the assumption by health professionals of responsibility for childbearing, which is implied in the risk approach, is desired by many people. Women who have the prospect of a normal birth but who nevertheless want birth in a consultant unit should have free access to such units, although they may not offer optimum safety and the best facilities for a normal birth.

We must understand birth in its simplicity, as something that is part of the conditions of human life.

CONCLUSION

Maternity care must be evaluated at various levels and in different ways. Evaluation should take as its starting point the questions asked by the users of the services. Any health service thus needs to have direct channels of communication with user organizations.

The use of different data bases for maternity care must take into account the fact that norms for laboratory values of normal births in consultant units are not necessarily identical with laboratory values for births where, for example, no drugs are given in labor.

Negative expectations for women's ability to be pregnant and to give birth are dangerous because they may become self-fulfilling prophecies. The experiences of midwives with spontaneous childbearing processes should be included as fundamental to the diagnosis and treatment of complicated and pathological processes.

Women and their families must be able to exercise real choice in the place of birth. This choice must be supported by knowledge and must not be limited by financial or other conditions. It should not cost anything, for example, to give birth in a consultant unit, even though a normal birth is anticipated.

A comprehensive and efficient system for adequate assistance in the home should be established for all births, where this is necessary or the woman or couple wants it. All births in institutions must take place according to the birthing woman's own conditions. Home birth in an institution is therefore a misleading concept, because a true birth at home differs from an institutional birth; the woman in her own home gives birth on her own territory.

If home birth is to yield good results, women and couples must genuinely desire their babies to be born at home. If this is not the case, they may feel so much insecurity that the birth process is disturbed, perhaps even complicated. The best results are achieved when birth attendants are also prepared for home birth and when they consider it in a positive light and not merely in terms of risks.

Normal pregnancies, births, and postpartum periods are the specialty of the midwife. Partly because of this, sufficient time needs to be set aside during prenatal care for the midwife and the woman to get to know each other.

The goal of maternity care is not limited to the prevention of morbidity and mortality and the establishment of secure conditions during pregnancy, birth, and the postpartum period. Beyond this, the goal is to give children a solid background for an adolescence and adulthood of which they and society can be proud, to give parents the best possible conditions in which to carry out the difficult and rewarding task of child-rearing, and to enable the professionals working in maternity services to provide the best, most sensitive, and least alienating care of which they are capable.

Chapter Seven

What Is Good Care?

Midwives and obstetricians are the major personal care providers for the child-bearing woman. They treat her, help her, and, they hope, support her through this important, rare, and special period in her life. For the woman, her care providers can assume an intimate importance she will remember for the rest of her life; what they do, what they say, and how they behave toward her, her baby, and her family may be unforgettable influences on her experience of becoming a mother. Her family, too, understand that the professionals attending her are important and may recall some of their sayings and doings a long time after the birth itself.

It is perhaps obvious that midwives and obstetricians believe that they give good care. They give the care they think is the best to obtain healthy babies after healthy pregnancies and normal births. What is good care? Opinions and practices differ. Outside the field of maternity care, there are large differences between countries, regions within the same country, and between different specialists in the use of common surgical procedures, such as appendectomy and tonsillectomy. Within obstetrics, use of technology, such as induction of labor, episiotomy, and Caesarean section, can vary threefold or fourfold. So individual practitioners have individual definitions of what constitutes good care. The basis of the definition may be an appeal to the lower mortality and morbidity believed to result from the practice in question; it may be local convenience or appropriateness; it may be habit. Each practitioner does in good faith what he or she believes to be right.

Yet although the different incidence of clinical procedures can be documented, there is relatively little evidence about the attitudes and opinions responsible for the differences. A study by Baruffi and others at Johns Hopkins University in the United States looked at the incidence of seven different obstetric procedures in two different institutions. Using a case control approach, they examined how similar groups of women were treated in the institutions. Matching these women's risk scores on a commonly used childbirth risk-scoring system with the treatment they actually received, the researchers found large differences between the two institutions. For example, 6 percent of low risk women received prenatal x rays in one institution, 16 percent in the other. During labor, the use of electronic fetal monitoring was 24 percent and 60 percent, respectively. Overall, the differences were greater, the lower the risk. The study's authors finally concluded that "the findings suggested that most of the differences did not reflect different levels of risk in the populations served, but were due to other unidentified factors."

Professionals, in general, are not particularly fond of being studied, and doctors are no exception to this rule. To find out more about the attitudes that shape these highly variable patterns of practice, and as part of our inquiry into the position of midwives in Europe today, we conducted interviews with obstetricians and midwives in four countries, two in northern Europe (Denmark and the United Kingdom) and two in southern Europe (Greece and Italy). The aim of these interviews was to explore ideas about good maternity care, in particular the notion of risk as applied to women having babies. Our interviews showed tremendous differences in the concept of good care. However, they had in common an underlying assumption that all professionals working in this field have in mind the best welfare of both mother and child. What is fascinating, therefore, is just how many different ways of managing pregnancy and birth can be constructed on this common ideological base.

The Sample of Midwives and Obstetricians

We interviewed forty-seven care-givers altogether: twenty-one obstetricians and twenty-six midwives (see Table 23 for some background information about our sample). The people we interviewed were not a random or representative sample. Using contacts we had in the different countries, we aimed to talk to roughly equal numbers of doctors and midwives and to achieve some spread between large and small hospitals and public versus private practice. Each of the midwives and obstetricians in our sample was given the same questions to

Table 23   The Midwives and Obstetricians in the Study

	The midwives (n = 26)	The obstetricians (n = 21)
Percentage female	100	19
Mean age	36 years	39 years
Mean number of children	1.5	1.8
Mean number of years in practice	14 years	12 years
Mean number of deliveries per year	80	86[a]
Percentage working wholly in private setting	27	14
Percentage working in urban areas	58	76

[a]Most of these were not actually done by the obstetrician but were supervised by him/her.

answer in the form of a standardized questionnaire. Some of the questions were open-ended and general, designed to elicit practitioners' views about actual and ideal birth services. Others took the form of vignettes or case stories for which we requested solutions. Some of our case stories concerned antenatal care, some the type of delivery that might be recommended in a particular case. We tried to put some social information as well as clinical facts into the stories, on the assumption that practitioners' responses might take account of this.

TALKING TO THE PROFESSIONALS

Before examining the responses, we present an excerpt from an interview with one of these care-givers, an obstetrician named Dr. Solomon, and an excerpt from an interview with a midwife. Dr. Solomon[1] is now working in a private clinic in the United Kingdom, having quite recently left a consultant post in a large hospital maternity unit.

> *Interviewer:* A twenty-eight-year-old woman is having her second child. She's twelve days overdue, according to dates and ultrasound, and the baby is estimated to weigh 3600 g. Her estriol levels are normal. Her first child weighed 3500 g and was delivered eight days after term. She has four and a half to five weeks in between her periods. What would you do?
>
> *Dr. Solomon:* I'd see her three times a week for that week, and then I'd see her every day after that. I would inform her that it was important for her to assess the baby's well-being by giving her some idea about fetal movements and fetal activity. I'd do an antenatal cardiograph, monitoring the fetal heart rate on alternate days for the first week, and then every day for the second week, and if it went on longer than that maybe even twice a day. We have a machine that people take home. They monitor it themselves.

[1]All names have been changed.

Interviewer: And do you scan the women?

Dr. Solomon: I don't believe that scanning has much to offer in terms of the planning of induction of labor.

Interviewer: So you'd look after her, but would you induce labor?

Dr. Solomon: Almost never. Unless there was an abnormality shown on the monitor, then I would start the labor off.

Interviewer: What is your emphasis during antenatal visits?

Dr. Solomon: They last half an hour, and the emphasis is technical and emotional. We do the blood pressure, maternal weight, urinalysis, and examination of the baby. And the emotional stuff just to find out what's been going on in her life, and to see whether there's anything we need to support her for, that she needs from us or that she needs other support from outside. We've got other support groups that I work quite closely with. We've got an acupuncturist, and sometimes for people who've got no energy, or pain, that can be very good. I work with an osteopath, particularly for backache and vomiting and headaches, and I also work with a psychotherapist. So we've got a good team.

Interviewer: The next story's about a twenty-six-year-old woman who's unmarried. She's living with a student and she's pregnant, having her first baby. She's been trying to get pregnant for two and a half years. She's twelve weeks pregnant now, and everything is normal. How would you treat her?

Dr. Solomon: She'll have her first antenatal visit, which will last approximately one hour, her full history will be taken, her past medical history, her gynecological history, with particular emphasis on her emotional life, her spiritual life, and nutrition, and any drugs, including alcohol and cigarettes. At this point, she'll meet the midwives, and she'll go on a tour of the unit, and she'll be shown where her baby's going to be born and introduced to the staff on the unit. She will then be given a handout inviting her to the mother and baby massage class and to the group discussions and the antenatal yoga sessions that happen each week. She'll be seen in the antenatal clinic every month up to twenty-eight weeks and then three-weekly, two-weekly, and weekly. If she goes past term, she'll be supervised three times a week or every day, and she'll have routine blood tests and an ultrasound scan at sixteen weeks, repeat hemoglobin and blood antibodies between thirty-two and thirty-six weeks. If there are any emotional, physical, or other problems that come up in the pregnancy, they're dealt with on an individual basis, the whole accent being on providing people with information and knowledge so that they feel confident to take care of themselves.

Interviewer: A thirty-one-year-old married teacher is having her first baby, and she wants a home delivery. No significant medical history, regular periods, certain about dates, planned pregnancy, nonsmoker, normal height and weight. Has had a normal pregnancy so far. Would you agree to a home delivery?

Dr. Solomon: I don't do home deliveries myself. But I often act as back-up for midwives who do do home deliveries. The answer to the question is yes, if a woman wants a home delivery, provided somebody is prepared to be present at the birth, I will offer back-up facilities for her.

Interviewer: What about antenatal care?

Dr. Solomon: What I frequently do is, when people are going to have a baby at home, I see them once in early pregnancy and I'll see them again around thirty-seven weeks or I'll see them in between at the request of the midwife.

Interviewer: A twenty-seven-year-old woman, a part-time secretary, had her first child three years ago after a pregnancy that was uncomplicated except for a weight gain of 23 kg and a rise in blood pressure to 145 over 100 just before delivery. Now she's pregnant again. She weighed 76 kg before this pregnancy and now, four weeks before term, she weighs 80 kg. Blood pressure 135 over 90. What kind of care would you advise?

Dr. Solomon: The first thing I would do is begin work to alter her diet, reducing sodium intake and fried foods. Basically a macrobiotic diet. Secondly, I would advise her to have acupuncture, because this can often bring down the blood pressure quite dramatically. Thirdly, I would advise her to have bed rest during the day of a few hours each day and to be seen in the antenatal clinic twice or three times a week. If the blood pressure continued to rise or if there was protein in the urine, or if there was any sign of fetal distress, then I would advise an induction of labor. However, depending on the condition of the baby, it may be necessary to perform a Caesarean section if it really got out of control.

Interviewer: The next one is a woman having her first baby, and she's certain of her dates. Obstetric conditions are favorable, and she asks for induction three days before her due date. No medical indication, but she wants induction so the baby will be born before her mother has to go back to Australia. What would you do in that situation?

Dr. Solomon: Terribly sorry, but the answer is no.

Interviewer: Next one is also about a home birth. A forty-year-old woman is having her fourth baby, and she's determined to have a home delivery. She's living in a cramped three-room apartment with the baby's father and her three other children, the two eldest by her ex-husband. The two eldest children are sixteen and fourteen years and were uncomplicated deliveries. The third child is two and a half now and was delivered by Caesarean. Labor began with ruptured membranes and had lasted twenty hours when the Caesarean was done. She has been strongly recommended to go to the obstetric unit, but refuses equally strongly. She says that, if no help is provided, she will give birth on her own.

Dr. Solomon: Well, I think it's everybody's right to do their own thing. I know that in this country the law's fairly specific and the maternity services have to support people in that sort of decision. And under those circumstances, yes, I would support the individual. But I think it's crazy. I think she's crazy.

Interviewer: Okay! The next one is a thirty-year-old primipara who goes into labor a few days past term. The delivery starts at home with ruptured membranes at six o'clock at night, and at eight o'clock she's in the hospital 2 cm dilated with clear amnion, the heartbeat is good, and there are no contractions. What would you do?

Dr. Solomon: How long have the membranes been ruptured?

Interviewer: Just for two hours.

Dr. Solomon: I would do a single vaginal examination to confirm the fact that the membranes are ruptured and to exclude the prolapse of the cord. I would then wait anything up to forty-eight hours before giving her drugs to stimulate uterine activity, as they almost always go into labor anyway. During this time, I would monitor for signs of infection in the uterus, particularly maternal temperature, pulse rate, and uterine tenderness. If the labor had not begun in forty-eight hours, I would start off labor using either intravenous syntocinon or vaginal prostaglandins.

Interviewer: The last one. A thirty-five-year-old woman having her third child. The dates are a bit unsure. She's in labor now, maybe two to four weeks early, although the midwife thinks she's at term. She has had three ultrasound scans that show she's maybe three to four weeks early. She's a smoker. She's in heavy labor when she comes into the ward. The dilatation is 6 cm. The membranes haven't ruptured. How would you treat her?

Dr. Solomon: (*Laughs.*) In the same way as I'd treat everybody else!

Interviewer: There's nothing wrong in that!

Dr. Solomon: She would be encouraged to have an active birth, we would perform fifteen minutes of continuous fetal heart monitoring, and provided the fetal heart was normal, she'd be encouraged to be up and about and active and mobile in labor. The fetal heart would be monitored intermittently every half-hour during the first stage and after every contraction during the second stage of labor; the membranes would not be ruptured unless there was either an abnormality on the fetal heart rate trace or, alternatively, there was prolongation of the first stage of labor.

Interviewer: What is the midwife's role in deliveries here? Are you there all the time or do you alternate with the midwives?

Dr. Solomon: We work as a team. We try to encourage the midwives who attend a woman in early labor to stay right through to the birth of the baby, and therefore the midwife and the woman are there virtually all the time together. And I kind of come and go. And usually stay continuously for the last two or three hours of the labor.

Interviewer: You know the woman beforehand; do the midwives have an opportunity to get to know her, too?

Dr. Solomon: Yes, the midwives come to every antenatal clinic.

Interviewer: How much does it cost to have a baby here?

Dr. Solomon: Do you want to know the total cost, including the obstetrician's fee?

Interviewer: Say I was a patient who came here, and I was twelve weeks pregnant, and I said I want to have care here, I want to have my delivery here?

Dr. Solomon: The cheapest would be about £400 and the average would be round about £1500.[2]

Interviewer: Okay. I want to ask you some questions about how you determine your treatment of women during pregnancy and delivery. When you see a woman in pregnancy, do you use categories of risk to determine what kind of problem she may encounter during the pregnancy and delivery?

Dr. Solomon: Yes, I have a risk chart that is part of the antenatal notes, but I don't have a risk score. I have a chart that says "risk factors," and they're categorized for me. I can show them to you if you like. (*Does so.*) All the notes have them. Past obstetric history–miscarriage risk, risk of intrauterine growth retardation, general medical problems.

---

[2]Rates quoted are those that were in effect in 1984.

Interviewer: That's something you've worked out yourself?

Dr. Solomon: Yes.

Interviewer: Do you include social factors in that?

Dr. Solomon: Yes, and emotional. Yes, very much so.

Interviewer: So when you have a woman in your clinic, how do you decide how to take care of her?

Dr. Solomon: Well, it depends on my assessment of her risk, on her needs, and our common decisions. That's how I decide.

Interviewer: So you also take care of her according to what she wants?

Dr. Solomon: Yes.

Interviewer: Do you take care of her according to your own subjective feeling of what is right?

Dr. Solomon: Very badly phrased question! Bad phrasing on that question. (*Laughs.*)

Interviewer: Okay, so what is your comment apart from that?

Dr. Solomon: According to my own subjective viewpoint? Sure, everybody treats people subjectively, but I try to be as relatively objective as possible.

Interviewer: Have you ever had any experience of using formal risk assessments?

Dr. Solomon: I certainly have! At the end of the day I think that it's important not to confine the obstetrician to risk scores. To leave the obstetrician and midwives the flexibility to get a feel for the individual rather than a risk score. I think risk scores are dangerous, because risk scores vary from year to year and fashion to fashion whereas gut feelings don't.

Interviewer: What is your attitude to a pregnant woman's own definition of risk?

Dr. Solomon: I take that very, very seriously, and I think that that's probably the most important risk category. Definitely. Here we get a lot of feedback from people because they're seen for half-hourly visits between twelve and sixteen times in the pregnancy—they've got eight hours—and they come every week, some of them, and we get very strong feelings about their own risk.

Interviewer: So you really believe in continuity of care?

Dr. Solomon: Oh God, yes. As you can see!

Interviewer: Do you agree with the routine use of ultrasound in pregnancy?

Dr. Solomon: I think it's quite useful at sixteen weeks, but if people have reservations about it then I certainly don't push it.

Interviewer: Do you feel that routine use of intrapartum electronic fetal heart monitoring reduces perinatal mortality?

Dr. Solomon: I think that the routine use of continuous electronic fetal heart monitoring increases the Caesarean section rate without reducing perinatal mortality. I think that if the electronic fetal heart monitor is used intermittently, the same way as midwives use the old-fashioned stethoscope, then it represents a major advance in intrapartum care.

Interviewer: Do you agree that pregnant women have a right to choose the kind of care they get? You've answered that really.

Dr. Solomon: Of course I do.

Interviewer: Do you think that women have an automatic right to abortion?

Dr. Solomon: (*Long pause.*) I think the Danes have got it right. Under twelve weeks, probably. Over twelve weeks, there has to be a bloody good reason to do it.

Interviewer: Is there anything you'd like to ask me?

Dr. Solomon: The only thing I want to add is that the way we practice here is the offshoot of a breakaway group of the Active Birth Movement, which focused attention on some of the problems of birth in the United Kingdom about two years ago. I then left the health service and came to work here, not because I object to the health service, I think it's fantastic, but because I needed to have a small family place. And this is what we've got here. I believe in continuity of care, and I don't believe in splitting pregnant women from women who've had their babies, I think that's ridiculous.

Interviewer: What kind of women do you find come here?

Dr. Solomon: Oh, middle-class people who can afford private care. But this is only an experimental group. It could be put into the community at very low cost.

Interviewer: Have you got any hard data?

Dr. Solomon: No, I've only been working here fifteen months; it's too soon for that.

A certain tension is detectable in this obstetrician's account of his approach to defining good care. He left the British National Health Service so as to provide better care; it is important to him that the care given by his team is holistic, including attention to diet, emotions, and the need for social support, and using alternative therapies such as acupuncture. He believes that women have a right to define their own care—indeed, he says this is the most essential element in his definition of risk. At the same time, he regards it as part of his task to inform women about such matters as fetal activity; it is his role to give them expert advice. He defends a woman's right to a home birth in one of the case stories, adding that he thinks she is crazy to do so (because of her past obstetric history). He does not, however, defend a woman's right to have an induction of labor if she so chooses. Even his defense of the right to home delivery is prefaced by a remark about the legal situation in the United Kingdom requiring the maternity services to provide care in such cases.

It is instructive to compare Dr. Solomon's responses to our questionnaire with those of Ms. Davey, an independent midwife practicing in the same city. Ms. Davey works as a community midwife in a London suburb. The first question Ms. Davey answers is the first Dr. Solomon was asked: a twenty-eight-year-old woman is having her second child, is now overdue, and a decision needs to be made about her care.

Ms. Davey: Apart from checking that she's well and doing the usual antenatal things—it'd be nice to see that she's still putting on weight and her blood pressure's normal, this kind of thing—I'd want to find out how she's feeling. Is she feeling okay about this? She's overdue, yes, but not worryingly overdue. Is there anything she can do to get things going herself? I would probably be saying, have you been making love recently? Discuss that with her. See if she's got any ideas. The fact that she's got a long cycle means she probably isn't overdue. Personally, I wouldn't be worried until she's about three weeks overdue. I think it might be reassuring to do something like a heart monitoring. I'd probably want to make sure that she knew the baby was moving and that she knew she could check that each day. Here most of the doctors—because it is the doctors who make the decisions—would be giving her a date for induction. And they certainly wouldn't give her the practical advice about how she might encourage things. I suppose they might also do an internal. But you were asking me what I would do as a midwife? I would be less worried about things like doing an internal to find out whether the cervix was ripe or not because, in a sense, what will that tell you?

Interviewer: The next one is a twenty-six-year-old woman, not married, living with a student, having her first baby. She's been trying to get pregnant for two and a half years; she's twelve weeks pregnant now, everything's normal. How would you treat her?

Ms. Davey: I think really—presumably she's got pregnant spontaneously without prolonged infertility treatment—I'd want to treat her as normal. She might be rather tense at first because it's taken her a long time to get pregnant, but she'd also be really, really excited. I'd like her to be able to relax a bit more. My advice would be, listen to your own body and its messages. You said she's unmarried, she's living with somebody—so she's got support there. I guess if he's a student they might be hard up. You can't tell; she might be working. But, again, you'd expect to discuss that—the kind of benefits and facilities that are available. At the beginning, it would be important to give her the chance to talk about what she wants and to give her the feeling that she's doing a healthy, normal thing.

Interviewer: What advice would you give about place of birth?

Ms. Davey: She should have the baby wherever she wants. It doesn't sound as though she's got any particular reason not to have a home delivery. In my experience, most women don't know about the options. I think possibly anybody who's got a positive wish to have a home delivery is a suitable case. There've certainly been occasions on which I've suggested a home delivery, but mostly by the time I meet women they've already decided to have the baby in hospital, and it isn't that aspect of their care they want to change.

Interviewer: The next one is a thirty-one-year-old married teacher who wants a home delivery. It's her first baby, she has no significant medical history, a planned pregnancy, regular periods, and is sure of her dates. She's a nonsmoker. Would you agree to a home delivery?

Ms. Davey: Yes.

Interviewer: Who should attend the birth?

Ms. Davey: Well, she could have whomever she wants. I think there should be a midwife there. Generally, the community midwives who do home deliveries teach student midwives, and, because there are so few home deliveries now, I think it's quite important to take a student. It teaches such a lot. I think it can give a student a whole different insight on the process of birth. You can't gain that in the same way in hospital because you're only seeing part of the process there.

Interviewer: What about antenatal care?

Ms. Davey: I don't think she needs extra antenatal care, but she might need different antenatal care . . . she might need some different guidance and preparation as regards the actual set-up for delivery.

Interviewer: Under what circumstances would you change her to a hospital booking?

Ms. Davey: Well, I think this is something you'd want to discuss with her at the outset before any problems arose. I think one problem that's picked up quite often, and which isn't often as serious as it seems, is intrauterine growth retardation. We often use technology in such a way that the process of pregnancy is not understood. We have a lot of women in the ward here who are told that their baby's too small, and they have to come into hospital. And then very often the distress of that makes the situation worse. Equally, there's an awful lot of overdiagnosis of the problem. So we haven't really learned how to use that technology to help women.

Interviewer: Do you use ultrasound routinely here?

Ms. Davey: Yes. We do it at sixteen and thirty-two weeks. If I was asked my opinion on that, I'd say that, if everything else had been normal and clinically the baby had been growing, I wouldn't particularly recommend a second scan because I think it often provides misleading information. It assumes that a baby grows at an even rate, which it doesn't. Growth is often related to things like stopping work, and, if you're doing the scan at that time, when the woman has only just stopped work, you're picking her up at a point where perhaps the baby hasn't been growing so fast. She stops work, has a couple of weeks' rest, and off it goes.

Interviewer: A twenty-seven-year-old married woman, working as a part-time secretary, is having her second child. Her first child was born three years ago following an uncomplicated pregnancy, except that she gained 23 kg and her blood pressure rose to 145 over 100. Her weight was 76 kg before this pregnancy, she's now thirty-six weeks, and her weight is 80 kg, her blood pressure 135 over 90. What would you say about the kind of care she ought to have?

Ms. Davey: She's really not put on half as much weight this time as she did last time. I'd obviously be checking carefully that she didn't have any proteinuria or any other signs of pre-eclampsia. I'd want to check to make sure she'd stopped work.

Interviewer: Can she stop work and not lose money?

Ms. Davey: Oh no, there's a terrible disincentive to stop work here. You must know how awful our maternity benefits are in this country? I think probably, if her first child was born three years ago, she wouldn't be covered by the contributions she'd paid before. So she probably wouldn't get maternity allowance just on that. If she's still working part-time, she might get maternity allowance—£25 a week roughly from twenty-eight weeks. So that would be a big drop in her pay. A lot of women choose to go on working because they have to. She's got a three-year-old as well; she's probably pretty tired. I'd want to see her resting more. If I detect any problem after twenty-eight weeks, it doesn't matter what the problem is, I immediately find out if they're still working and discuss that with them because the state does technically allow them to stop working at twenty-eight weeks. They don't lose their job security or their maternity rights.

Interviewer: A woman having her first baby, who's sure of her dates, wants an induction three days before her due date so that the baby will be born before her mother goes back to Australia. Obstetric conditions are favorable. What would you do?

Ms. Davey: That's difficult. It's very difficult. It would be against my better judgment, but her wishes are very important. I would be quite worried about her situation, because interfering without good cause is likely to run into problems. We could assess the cervix first of all, see if it was favorable. I guess if it was favorable, and it looked as if it would be a straightfoward induction, perhaps I .would feel less unhappy about it. I can't say I would be overjoyed. Without trying to scare her, I think I would present her with information about what was involved. I think it is important, if somebody has chosen people to be with them, that that should be possible, but I can't help feeling that it is such an important thing that the mother should be a bit more flexible. I do believe in a woman's right to choose in every circumstance, and would be prepared to let the mother take a decision as long as I was happy that she understood it.

Interviewer: Right, now we have a forty-year-old woman having her fourth baby, and she wants a home delivery. She's living in a cramped three-room apartment with the baby's father and her three other children, the two eldest by her ex-husband. The two eldest children are sixteen and fourteen years and were uncomplicated deliveries. The third child is two and a half now and was delivered by Caesarean. Labor began with ruptured membranes and had lasted twenty hours when the Caesarean was done. She has been strongly recommended to go to the obstetric unit, but refuses equally strongly. She says that, if no help is provided, she will give birth on her own.

Ms. Davey: You don't get anywhere by frightening people or being negative. I think I would want to make sure at the beginning that she does understand she has a right to home delivery, and she would be cared for by us there, which she would be, certainly in this area. I think the Caesarean scar would perhaps be more worrying than her age and her parity. I think, once somebody feels you're on their side, then they're more prepared to trust you. It would hopefully be possible to build up a relationship with her, so that you could say, look, these are the worries we have, and she wouldn't think you were just trying to put her off a home delivery. It could be that a compromise would be acceptable—for example, a domino delivery, whereby a community midwife who'd got to know her in pregnancy could bring her into hospital, deliver her, and take her home again. This could be an acceptable compromise, but if it wasn't, then we'd deliver her at home. I think in those circumstances I'd want another midwife there, and I'd quite like there to be a doctor available. One other point, something we don't do in this country, as midwives we're not really taught how to put up intravenous infusions. As community midwives, you don't necessarily carry that equipment, so that would be something to bear in mind.

Interviewer: A thirty-year-old primipara is in labor a few days past term. Labor begins with ruptured membranes at six o'clock at night, and at eight o'clock she's in the hospital 2 cm dilated with clear amnion, the heartbeat is good, and there are no contractions. What would you do?

Ms. Davey: I'd see if she's had any food, make sure she gets her supper and hope she gets a good night's sleep! (*Laughs.*) Once her membranes have ruptured, then really labor's got to happen. I think if in the morning there hadn't been any action—if we'd done an internal, we would have tried to stir things up a bit—we might even consider something like an enema. I'd assume she'd want to avoid a drip; well, I would want to avoid a drip.[3] I might encourage her to get up and walk around in the morning. Then after a few hours, and obviously keeping an eye on the fetal heart and the temperature, she'd have to have syntocinon. But basically what we'd hope is that during the night she'd go into labor!

Interviewer: Finally, the last story: a thirty-five-year-old woman having her third child is in heavy labor; her dates are a little unsure, maybe two to four weeks early, although the midwife thinks she's at term. She has had three ultrasound scans that show she's maybe three to four weeks early. She's a smoker. When she comes into the ward, the dilatation is 6 cm. The membranes haven't ruptured. How would you treat her?

Ms. Davey: Well, she's obviously going to deliver. I'd want to monitor the heartbeat continuously. I think she's at risk of having a baby that's growth-retarded; I won't rely on the scan, but I won't ignore that information: it fits with her smoking. I certainly would want to check that everything was going normally. I might even quite like a pediatrician around for the delivery. For some reason, I feel there are going to be problems here. I guess I would consider rupturing the membranes if she didn't have any strong feelings against that.

Interviewer: Do you use predetermined categories of risk in deciding the kind of care someone would have?

Ms. Davey: Yes, but I don't categorize people as just high risk and low risk. It's not as simple as that. I think you're looking at a whole lot of different factors, and you're forming a picture in your own mind of this individual woman and her situation, and you also often do get impressions and feelings about somebody that you can't always put into a definite category. I base my treatment on any definite information I've got—any tests and investigations—on what the woman says, on what I know about her and her social situation, and also, as I said, my own feeling about somebody.

Interviewer: So you take into account your own subjective feelings about her?

Ms. Davey: I think it relates to how a woman's feeling about herself. If she's feeling tense, this often comes over, and it says to me, here's somebody who might be tense about giving birth, and I'd like to help her relax a bit. If she finds it difficult to relax, maybe she's more at risk of having high blood pressure, and so on. Or it often relates to somebody who's looking very tired. You can spot that, and you think, is she eating okay, is she having problems sleeping, has she got home problems? But there are people who have special medical histories who do need to see the consultant. They may not be suitable for general practitioner care, let alone midwife care.

Interviewer: And do you give a woman the kind of care she wants?

Ms. Davey: To a certain extent. But then I also think that, particularly with a first pregnancy, you don't always know what you want. As a midwife, you need to

[3]*Drip:* Intravenous drugs to induce labor.

have a certain standard of education and sharing of information with a woman, even if she doesn't always take the initiative in asking for it.

Interviewer: I think you've already answered the question as to whether you use your own subjective feelings in deciding care, haven't you?

Ms. Davey: I do use them to a certain extent. I'm not totally disregarding the limits of our practice, I am aware of those, I am aware of what constitutes a problem, what constitutes high risk, what constitutes a medical complication, but I think the woman herself needs to understand as much as possible so that what she wants will be appropriate. If she has no information, she can't make a decision.

Interviewer: Do you take into account her own definition of risk?

Ms. Davey: I think either way round, it always means something. In my experience, if a woman comes to you and says something's wrong, then you'd better jolly well listen! A lot of problems are missed that way. Women's instincts tell them all sorts of things; there are instances where everyone—the consultant and everyone—has assured a woman nothing's wrong, and she has actually proved to be right, and the baby is abnormal. So I suppose one's got to be careful not to be too dogmatic and categorical. The other aspect, when you know there's a problem and she won't accept it or believe it, the problem is her attitude: she needs to be helped to accept it. It isn't easy; it is threatening, to accept some complication, and you need to discuss what she thinks it means—often people have heard things that aren't true. Let's say the baby is a breech, and friends have told her it'll therefore have to be a Caesarean, and she doesn't want to accept the baby's breech, but what she really doesn't want is a Caesarean. So you've got to find out what it is that she doesn't accept and then work her through that to face up to the problem.

Interviewer: Do you agree with routine ultrasound?

Ms. Davey: No.

Interviewer: Do you think that the routine use of continuous electronic fetal heart rate monitoring reduces perinatal mortality?

Ms. Davey: I don't know. If you're asking for my feelings, no, I don't think it does. But I don't have evidence, though there's no evidence that I've seen that it does.

Interviewer: Do you think pregnant women have a right to choose the kind of care they get?

Ms. Davey: Yes.

Interviewer: Do you think women have an automatic right to abortion?

Ms. Davey: Yes!

DEFINING GOOD CARE

The similarities and the differences between these accounts are almost equally fascinating. Both Dr. Solomon and Ms. Davey emphasize the importance of taking women's own perspectives and the totalities of their situations into account in deciding what constitutes good care in any individual case. One is nevertheless led to understand that, for Dr. Solomon, this principle represents acceptance at the ideological level of the importance of user-sensitive care, rather than a thorough attempt to consider what the principle might mean in everyday practice. For example, when asked if he would consider inducing a woman because she herself wants an induction, Dr. Solomon immediately says no. Ms. Davey, on the other hand, expresses her feeling that this situation is very difficult, and necessitates balancing her professional judgment as a midwife with the mother's right to have at the birth those support people of her choice, and in general to exercise her right to choose at all times. In the end, she concludes that it is her duty as a midwife to give information about the hazards of induction and that, if the mother still wants induction, she should then be allowed the responsibility of taking this decision.

In general, Dr. Solomon is more prone than Ms. Davey to consider first the monitoring and intervention techniques that might be appropriate for the women in our case stories. He is not happy at the suggestion that his subjective feelings about a woman might influence the type of care she ought to be given. In contrast, Ms. Davey links the value she attaches to these feelings in herself with the probability that they reflect something she has picked up from the woman herself.

Tables 24–31 show samples of reactions to the case stories from both midwives and doctors in our sample. As we said, our sample is small, and not selected at random, so it is not possible to generalize from it. However, the responses do offer some clues as to how the attitudes and practices of midwives may differ in systematic ways from those of obstetricians.

Table 24 concerns the woman with the weight gain problem that might be prejudicial to the pregnancy. Dr. Solomon's response—to advise diet, acupuncture, and bed rest—seems more constructive than that of the obstetrician who says he would be angry because the patient is "out of control." It is interesting that the midwife takes a quite authoritarian line ("she should do whatever the obstetrician tells her").

Table 25 poses a question about delivery policies. What do midwives and obstetricians feel about a woman who is in fairly advanced labor but whose membranes are intact? Is her smoking relevant? What about the uncertainty concerning the baby's gestational age? The first obstetrician to answer this is interesting: he begins by saying he would treat her as normal and then goes on to say that he'd "like" to rupture the membranes: "I'd like to see the color of the water, and what's going on" (Ms. Davey also expressed an interest in rupturing the membranes, although in a different way). The second doctor flatly refuses to believe the midwife instead of the ultrasound so far as the dates are concerned. The third one from Italy spells out a list of drugs and other procedures that could be used in this case; his mind moves quickly to what can be done technologically rather than perhaps what this case merits. The fourth doctor picks up on the issue of maternal smoking, but he's not quite sure what this means clinically. The next response, from a midwife, uses the cliché of letting nature take its course and likens the fetal image on the ultrasound screen to an unidentified flying object.

Table 24 Case Study: Pregnancy with Weight Gain

		Recommendations from care-givers (summarized)			
Case	Obstetrician, United Kingdom	Midwife, Greece	Obstetrician, Greece	Obstetrician, United Kingdom	Obstetrician, United Kingdom
A 27-year-old married woman, a part-time secretary, had her first child 3 years ago following a pregnancy that was uncomplicated except for a weight gain from 62 to 85 kg and a rise in blood pressure to 145 over 100 just before delivery. Weight 76 kg before this pregnancy; now at 36 weeks, weight 80 kg, blood pressure 135 over 90. What kind of care would you advise for her now?	We'd probably see her in the consultant unit and do serial uric acid measurements each week. If these don't rise and she doesn't develop proteinuria and the uric acids are okay, we'd leave her. We'd probably do human placental lactogens as well, because the chances are that I'd see her every week. She'll be asked to rest, and we'd get one of our girls to phone up for a community midwife, who will go to the home to check the patient twice a week.	She should do whatever the obstetrician tells her, take the medicine he'll prescribe for her blood pressure, and a little before her due date come in for an induction.	I'd be very angry because of her weight gain. She's a high-risk patient because she's out of control.	First, I would convince her to have antenatal care more often: every 14 days, and then once a week at the end. I would not hospitalize her at this stage.	The first thing I'd do is begin work to alter her diet. Secondly, I would advise her to have acupuncture to bring down her blood pressure. Thirdly, I would advise her to have bed rest during the day and be seen in the antenatal clinic 2 or 3 times a week. If the blood pressure continued to rise or if there was protein in the urine or there was any sign of fetal distress, then I would advise an induction of labor. It might be necessary to perform a Caesarean section if it really got out of control.

147

Table 25 Case Study: Delivery Policies

	Recommendations from care-givers (summarized)				
Case	Obstetrician, Denmark	Obstetrician, Italy	Obstetrician, Italy	Obstetrician, Greece	Midwife, Denmark
A 35-year-old woman is having her third child. The dates are a bit unsure. She might be in labor now, 3–4 weeks early. She has had 3 ultrasound scans that show that she is maybe 3–4 weeks early, but the midwife's opinion is that she's at term. She is a smoker. She is in heavy labor when she comes into the ward, the dilatation is 6 cm, the membranes haven't ruptured. How would you treat this woman?	I'd just treat her as normal. I would warn the special care unit that we've got a case, a bit early. I think If she's 6 cm I'd like to rupture the membranes. I'd like to see the color of the water and what's going on.	I can't believe the midwife more than the ultrasound; after all, she's coming to me to ask for help, I must make the interpretation.	If the cervix is 6 cm, we could give her cortisone in case the infant is premature. Then leave her quietly overnight in the hospital to see what happens. We could give her a tranquilizer. Later we could break the water artificially and give oxytocin and have a special care baby unit stand by. The fact that she smokes could account for the small size of the baby.	How many cigarettes a day does she smoke? If a woman smokes in pregnancy 2 things could apply: first, the baby really is full-term and, because she smokes, it has a lower birth weight, or a mistake has happened and the baby is premature. We could rupture the membranes or we could wait a bit and let things go on as they are.	Let nature take its course. Ultrasound is done by technicians, not doctors. It must have been done for some particular reason. No mother-to-be wants to see her infant as a UFO.

Table 26 Case Study: Whether or Not to Intervene

			Recommendations from care-givers (summarized)			
Case	Midwife, United Kingdom	Midwife, Italy	Midwife, United Kingdom	Midwife, Denmark	Obstetrician, Italy	Obstetrician, United Kingdom
A 30-year-old primipara goes into labor a few days past term. Labor starts with ruptured membranes at 6 p.m. At 8 p.m., she is in hospital. She is only dilated about 2 cm. Clear amnion, heartbeat good. No contractions. What would you do from here?	I wouldn't have her in the hospital anyway. I'd just leave her, I wouldn't do an internal, no nothing. The danger of infection is very little at home anyway. So long as the amnion is clear, I'd let her wait several days.	We wait 24 hours, but she must take antibiotics and see the doctor. After that we induce.	I'd see if she has had any food, make sure she got her supper, and hope she gets a good night's sleep. If in the morning there hadn't been any action—if we'd done an internal, we would have tried to stir things up a bit—we might even consider an enema. I'd assume she'd want to avoid a drip; well, I would want to avoid a drip. I might encourage her to get up and walk around in the morning. Then after a few hours she'd have to have syntocinon.	I'd ask how she felt—if she was tired or if she was quite fit. I'd give her a massage and see if it caused any contractions. If by midnight she didn't have any, I'd let her sleep. We would have to induce her in the morning.	If contractions haven't begun after 6 hours, I'd induce. If the first drip doesn't induce, I'd wait 6 hours and give a second. It's absolutely necessary to give antibiotics, and we must do a culture to make sure there aren't any pathological microbes in the vagina to begin with.	I'd probably let her walk around for a while. They have a bath, and if they haven't had their bowels open that day, they get a course of suppositories. You don't normally give enemas, and you don't shave them either. I'd encourage her to walk about, and I'd feed her to give the uterus something to work on, and then I'd just wait and see what happens. If after 12 hours she hadn't done very much, then we'd offer her some syntocinon. But again if they refuse (they don't usually refuse if you talk to them sensibly), the longer you leave them with the waters gone, the more risk there is to the baby.

149

Table 27 Case Study: History of Infertility

Case	Midwife, United Kingdom	Obstetrician, Greece	Obstetrician, Italy	Midwife, Denmark	Midwife, United Kingdom	Obstetrician, Italy
			Recommendations from care-givers (summarized)			
A 26-year-old single woman living with a student is pregnant for the first time following 2-1/2 years of infertility. At 12 weeks, everything is normal. How would you treat her during pregnancy and birth?	I wouldn't consider her as being at risk because I feel it's quite normal not to become pregnant straight away; also, she's under 30. I'd try to find out how she has lived in those 2-1/2 years: has she had a stable relationship, or has she just wished to get pregnant and lived with different men? Has she really tried to plan her pregnancy? I think I would treat her quite normally. I'd let her have the normal examinations, and if there were complications I'd ask her to contact us straight away, but I'd also say that to anyone else.	As it has been difficult for her to become pregnant, I would expect some difficulties. I'd probably have her admitted to hospital in the last 2 weeks of the pregnancy.	It's a good question. We'd have to do very careful examinations, hormone tests, estriols, also urine cultures and blood tests. Also, we'd look out for any bleeding or discharge or early contractions. She'll probably have a forceps delivery. If there are any problems, then we'll decide on a C-section. Because of the history of infertility, we might have problems, even *placenta praevia* or *abruptio*.	As usual. Now the problem is over, she is pregnant and that is probably a sign of health.	As a community midwife, I don't think I'd treat her really any differently. She's the sort of person who might appreciate home visits because she might need the extra reassurance and time. Because she has been infertile, she's likely to be more anxious. What she needs is just time to talk. She needs to be advised exactly what the services are, what to expect.	I'd like her extra antenatal care. In the presence of the slightest risk, I'd perform a C-section.

Table 28 Case Study: Induction (Postterm)

Case	Obstetrician, Italy	Obstetrician, Italy	Midwife, Greece	Midwife, Italy	Midwife, Denmark	Midwife, United Kingdom
		Recommendations from care-givers (summarized)				
A 28-year-old woman having her second baby is 12 days overdue according to dates and ultrasound. Baby's weight is estimated at 3600 g. Human placental lactogens and estriol levels are normal. Hormone tests are okay. Her first child weighed 3500 g and was delivered at term + 8 days. Her menstrual cycle is 4-1/2–5 weeks. What should be done?	I'd wait until 42 weeks and then I'd do an induction. Meanwhile, I'd give her a kick chart and an amnioscopy every day. I don't take any notice of the menstrual cycle if I have 2 ultrasound scans.	I wouldn't have let this pregnancy go over the due date by so many days. We'd have to do a series of tests to be sure the infant is mature first and then induce. After all, we're dealing with a case of potential stillbirth.	As a midwife in Greece, I don't have the right to do anything in this case. I'd send the woman to the doctor, and he'll say what has to be done. I wouldn't induce labor. It's up to the doctor.	If there's some dilatation of the cervix, I'd suggest an amnioscopy. If the amniotic fluid is clear, I'd wait 2 more days. Then I'd admit her to hospital so as to attempt oxytocic stimulation.	First of all, I'd see how she felt psychologically and physically at this stage. Then I'd study her first pregnancy: time of delivery, if she was overdue then, too. Then I'd go back to the ultrasound and do a new calculation, remembering her long cycle. She'd be just about due now. I'd send her to the doctor next time because, according to our directives, she must see the doctor at 41 weeks.	I'd check that she is well, still gaining weight, blood pressure normal, etc. I'd suggest that maybe making love might push things on a bit or even a dose of castor oil. She's not too much overdue, and it probably has something to do with her long menstrual cycle. A doctor at this stage would be more inclined to give a date for induction after doing an internal examination, but I'd be inclined to let the mother go longer and encourage the mother to do something herself.

Table 29 Case Study: Induction on Request

			Recommendations from care-givers (summarized)			
Case	Obstetrician, Greece	Midwife, Denmark	Midwife, Italy	Obstetrician, Denmark	Midwife, United Kingdom	Obstetrician, Italy
A woman having her first baby is certain of her dates. Obstetric conditions are favorable, and she asks for induction 3 days before her expected date of delivery. There are no medical indications, but she wants induction so that the baby will be born before her mother has to go back to Australia. What would you advise her to do?	I would send her elsewhere; I'd absolutely say no to this. I never like to go against nature.	I'd wonder why it's so important for her to have her mother around, and I'd talk to her about it. I know there will be trouble if you induce. But, of course, she could try one of the natural methods.	I'm sorry, but I just don't think you should mess around like that, although I do sympathize. But I think she'd be mad to ask to be induced. If she was very insistent and if it was going to mean so much to her, given the fact that they induce so many people anyway for all sorts of very strange reasons, I think the mother should probably have the choice. I certainly wouldn't advise it.	I'd advise her not to be induced. I'd tell her that the risk of complications is higher. It's very seldom that I meet women like this—maybe some years ago, but not now. If it were some kind of difficult social problem, I'd be much more open to induction.	I can understand her feelings. I'd examine her internally, and if the cervix was very ripe, then I'd try to get it done. Otherwise, I wouldn't want to deal with it!	We must follow physiology. Every induction is risky. It must be done only if it is worth it. I don't agree with induction.

Table 30 Case Study: Home Birth (Fourth Baby)

Case	Midwife, United Kingdom	Midwife, Greece	Recommendations from care-givers (summarized) Obstetrician, Greece	Obstetrician, Italy	Obstetrician, Italy	Midwife, United Kingdom
A 40-year-old woman having her fourth baby is determined to have a home delivery. She lives in a cramped 3-room apartment with the baby's father and 3 other children (the 2 eldest by her ex-husband). The 2 eldest children are 16 and 14 years and were uncomplicated deliveries. The third child, 2-1/2, was delivered by Caesarean. Labor began with ruptured membranes and had lasted 20 hours when the Caesarean was done. She has been counseled to go into the local obstetric unit, but refused strongly. She says if no help can be provided, she will give birth on her own! What would you advise her to do?	I see no problem at all. I see no reason at all why she shouldn't have her baby at home. I don't think her age makes any difference.	If she calls me when she's in labor, I'd go as quickly as possible and try to get her into hospital. I wouldn't want her to deliver at home. In the end, she'd go into hospital, the whole village would persuade her to, and her husband would, too.	I would send the police to get her. If I knew beforehand, I'd send the police; I would probably go along, too. If I didn't know beforehand, I would go.	I'd send her to a psychiatrist. If she really insisted, I'd follow her at home, but I'd want an ambulance ready.	I wouldn't want to be her doctor unless she paid me a lot.	I'd look for a midwife with many years of experience. I'd call the hospital, explain the case, and ask to have doctor available if needed. I'd look at the medical records of the third baby to see the indication and description of the Caesarean section.

153

Table 31 Case Study: Home Birth (First Baby)

Case	Obstetrician, United Kingdom	Obstetrician, Italy	Obstetrician, United Kingdom	Midwife, Italy	Midwife, Greece	Midwife, Italy
			Recommendations from care-givers (summarized)			
A 31-year-old married teacher having her first baby wants a home delivery. No significant medical history. Regular periods. Certain about dates. Planned pregnancy. Nonsmoker, 1.72 m tall, weight 62 kg before pregnancy. Normal pregnancy. Would you agree to a home delivery?	I wouldn't agree to home delivery because she's a teacher, and generally teachers are very anxious.	No home delivery. I wouldn't take the responsibility. It takes too much time. I don't have enough experience, and I wouldn't know how to organize it. However, if she paid me a lot of money, I would do it.	I'd agree to a home delivery if the risk score indicates a normal birth. I am in favor of home birth when women so desire and the prognosis is for a normal birth.	No home delivery. In each birth, we can face lots of problems, e.g., hemorrhoids, maybe *placenta praevia*, maybe the infant will need extra care. It's just better to do it in the hospital. Maybe the placenta won't separate as it should.	If she'd been in hospital during the pregnancy for observation because of the baby not growing as it should or if the hormone levels were below normal, I'd try to talk her out of delivery at home; also, considering her age, if she develops low blood pressure or problems during pregnancy.	No. At home, there's no equipment, and it isn't the right environment to give birth in.

154

The next question (Table 26) introduces similar dilemmas about interventionist versus noninterventionist philosophies. The problem here is the absence of contractions after a spontaneous rupture of the membranes. One midwife baldly states that the best thing to do is not to have the mother in the hospital: the risk of infection is much less at home. Still, she feels she'd like to see if she can stimulate contractions. A second midwife recites hospital policy—a wait of twenty-four hours during which the mother is given antibiotics, then induction. The third midwife, Ms. Davey, assumes that both mother and midwife would wish to avoid an artificially accelerated labor if possible. The fourth takes the line that the mother should be looked after, should get some sleep, and so on, but the midwife would probably try to get the contractions started.

The two obstetricians take somewhat different sides on this case. The first is very specific about what he would do: induce after six hours. He would give antibiotics, and he suspects the mother of harboring pathogens in her vagina. His colleague would let the woman walk around for a while, eventually offering syntocinon. Note, however, that he slips from talking about "she" to saying "they." He classes this individual woman along with other women like her, so far as advising his particular desired course of action is concerned, and somewhat patronizingly remarks that "they don't usually refuse if you talk to them sensibly."

One of our case stories invites the professionals providing care for pregnant women to consider the relevance of a history of infertility (Table 27). One midwife queries the diagnosis, pointing out that a delay in conceiving is probably normal anyway. Another midwife simply counts the label as irrelevant. Yet a third, who works in the community, considers she does have special needs because of her history, but these are for reassurance rather than intensive clinical monitoring. All three obstetricians, by contrast, advise heightened clinical care. Two mention a Caesarean section, and one, antenatal hospital admission.

However, it is when we come to the hot issues of induction and home birth—especially the latter—that this group of midwives and obstetricians most clearly divide themselves into separate camps. The first of the two case stories concerning induction presents a woman, otherwise normal, who is twelve days past her due date (Table 28). The second asks the question, would you consider doing an induction on purely social grounds because the woman herself wants it (Table 29)?

In the first case, the issue is deliberately complicated because the question includes mention of the woman's naturally prolonged menstrual cycle. In questions of induction, accurate dating of the pregnancy is of paramount importance. Does the best care consist of trusting the information gleaned from ultrasound scans or from the patient herself? The first obstetrician categorically asserts, "I don't take any notice of the menstrual cycle if I have two ultrasound scans." The second obstetrician also quite categorically asserts that he wouldn't have let the pregnancy go past its due date by so many days anyway. The midwives are divided. The one from Greece does not regard herself as having the professional right to make a decision, so she is let off the hook. The next one adopts a cautious attitude, bringing up the question of the state of the woman's cervix and being prepared to wait two days if everything seems all right. The remaining two midwives give longer answers. They refer to the mother's general condition. One goes back to the question of dates, does a recalculation, allowing for the woman's long cycle, and decides she's only just about due now; however, at 41 weeks, she must be sent to the doctor because local directives say so. Her colleague also refers to the probability that the woman is not really overdue and goes on to recommend more natural methods of induction—intercourse and/or castor oil—than oxytocin.

If midwives and obstetricians are sometimes willing to induce on the basis of suspicion of an overdue baby, how do they feel about being asked to do so for the mother's personal convenience? None of them are prepared to say yes to this, although one midwife wavers and ends up by deciding that, especially in view of prevailing induction policies, the mother should probably have the choice. She admits that if the woman's cervix is "ripe" she'd try to do it for her. It may be difficult to believe the obstetrician who says, "I never like to go against nature," or his colleague who remarks, "We must follow physiology," since it seems unlikely that they fit the rest of their practices entirely around these precepts. Indeed, each contradicts himself on this point in the other answers he gives to the questionnaire. The second obstetrician says he might do what a woman wants if a difficult social problem is involved. A return ticket for one's mother to Australia apparently is not a difficult social problem; it appears that the doctor must be included in the business of defining exactly what would be one. Finally, one midwife takes up the question of why the woman feels it is so important to have her mother around. And how about—once again—natural methods of induction in preference to artificial ones?

Two women in our hypothetical series wanted a home birth. One, aged forty years, is having her fourth baby (Table 30); one, aged thirty-one years, is having her first (Table 31). Our forty-year-old came in for some harsh comments. One doctor would send her to a psychiatrist; another would call the police. The obstetrician, Dr. Solomon, quoted earlier called her crazy. Another obstetrician, from Italy, showed his practical side: "I wouldn't want to be her doctor unless she paid me a lot." Cultural differences are exposed in the answer given by the Greek midwife, who summons up the persuasive powers of the entire village to get the mother into the hospital. Another midwife merely sees no problems. A third is the only one to make the intelligent suggestion of reviewing the case notes of the third baby to find out more about the reasons why a Caesarean section was done.

The younger woman receives slightly more sympathetic treatment from our sample, although one midwife does refer to her age as an indication for "talking her out" of a home delivery. The phrase "I'd try to talk her out of it" does, however, convey a qualitatively different attitude from the others, who use terms such as "risk score" or cite the well-known occupational anxiety of the teaching profession as a contraindication to home birth. One obstetrician (from Italy) complains he is unable to take the responsibility of a home birth; he lacks experience and would not know how to organize it anyway. In the end, he reveals himself to be a pragmatic chap: "If she pays me a lot of money, I would do it."

PRACTICAL AND PROFESSIONAL LIMITS

In general, the obstetricians in our small study are more concerned about pathology than the midwives; twice as many midwives as doctors articulated the assumption that pregnancy and birth are normal processes, and that it should be the job of the people providing care to ensure that this inherent normality is translated into reality. The following tests or interventions were significantly more favored by obstetricians than midwives in their accounts of how they would treat the cases we asked them about: antenatal cardiography, nonstress tests, ultrasound scanning, electronic fetal heart rate monitoring, tests of placental function, internal examinations, and induction of labor. When asked whether they approved of routine ultrasound in pregnancy, 70 percent of midwives said no, compared with 33 percent of obstetricians. A question about the possible contribution of continuous electronic fetal heart rate monitoring to reducing perinatal mortality produced a similar but smaller professional divide, with 39 percent of doctors and 50 percent of midwives disclaiming any connection. Almost all these methods of care were recommended more often in Greece and Italy than in Denmark or the United Kingdom. In general, the Greek and Italian obstetricians were more inclined to favor technology and inflexible rules than their counterparts in Denmark and the United Kingdom. Alternative or, rather, traditional methods of intervention, such as sexual intercourse, nipple stimulation, castor oil, acupuncture, and homeopathy, were all likely to be mentioned by midwives and not by obstetricians. Between-country differences were also evident in some of the midwives' responses; the Greek and Italian midwives more clearly deferred to doctors' judgments than did their more independent-minded sisters in northern Europe.

The general predisposition among professionals providing maternity care to terminate the processes of pregnancy and labor is perhaps hardly surprising. Among the obstetricians, the northern doctors were much more relaxed about this than their southern colleagues. Aside from local differences in definitions of midwife autonomy, there were no parallel divisions among the midwives. One illustration of this is the possible use of artificial rupture of the membranes in the question we asked about the woman who entered hospital in heavy labor but with intact membranes; almost all the southern doctors would rupture her membranes, whereas their northern peers tended to adopt a wait-and-see attitude. In each country, half the midwives would rupture the membranes and half would not do so.

The midwives' answers tended to say a great deal about the extent of autonomy they were able to experience in their work situations. One British midwife, for instance, responding to the assertive woman in our case story who wanted an induction, began to describe her own reaction, then stopped herself: "It's unfortunate, but I'm not terribly (laughs)! Anyway, that in actual fact is a doctor's decision, and they would probably say all right, we'll do it. That's up to them. I wouldn't touch it, no, I would not! It's not up to the midwives to make those sorts of decisions, not at all! . . . I'm very much for the midwife's role, but, once you start going outside your role, it's not professional, it is?"

What is professional in one place is not so in another. For the midwife, the limits of her professional practice are set not only by the internal standards of her own profession but by others, and particularly by what obstetricians in specific institutional settings think she should be allowed to do.

A midwife's reluctance to become involved in the patient's rights, as seen in the example just quoted, highlights the attitude of some midwives, who wish to stay within a limited version of their role, not to step outside it. Similarly, not all the midwives display an awareness of the importance of social factors. Discussing the case of the student with a history of infertility, one said, "If she's a single girl living with a student, she's going to need psychological as well as physical care. She'll need all the ancillary services, she'll need to have those brought to her attention." Of course, it may be that this woman's personal situation does leave her vulnerable and in need of help from social workers and others, but it is hardly fair to assume this. Compare this answer with Ms. Davey's answer to the same case story.

Differences between obstetricians and midwives do, to some extent, reflect their different working situations. Among the doctors we interviewed, none did home births, one worked in a birth center, seven in an ordinary hospital with a birth room, and thirteen in hospital-based maternity units. Among the midwives, two were exclusively involved in home births, three combined this with some hospital practice, four worked in conventional hospitals with birth rooms, nine practiced in hospital-based maternity units, and four worked in maternity homes. In Denmark, pregnant women see a doctor only once antenatally unless complications develop. In the United Kingdom, all pregnant women see doctors, although midwives are also responsible for a good deal of antenatal care. In Greece and Italy, midwives are not involved in taking responsibility for antenatal care at all, except when they practice privately, undertaking home deliveries.

Denmark is the only one of the four countries to have official risk-scoring guidelines, published by the Ministry of Health. Elsewhere, practice differs, both officially and unofficially. Yet it is significant that all the care-givers we talked to spontaneously mentioned the term risk; only when they were asked to spell out what they meant did the different meanings of the term become apparent. From obstetricians who always use a predetermined list of medical and obstetric risk factors to shape the care they offer in individual cases, the spectrum of meanings extends to midwives who talk about the need to feel good about the women they look after. A couple of midwives observed that red hair always spells problems; Greek midwives were, for some reason, especially prone to mention personal appearance as an important indicator of risk! One obstetrician who was quite inflexible about some of his definitions of risk—for instance, he would not grant the primigravida in our case story the right to a home birth because "I think all primigravidas of whatever age should be delivered in hospital"—went on to explain the somewhat tenuous basis of these judgments he makes about risk:

> *Doctor:* We don't use a formal risk system. We're talking about it at the moment. We use a qualitative method—we might well write down "high risk" without counting any score up.
> *Interviewer:* Then does everyone know what "high risk" is?
> *Doctor:* No, you're absolutely right, no. I might write down why I think they're high risk: previous stillbirth or whatever. But that doesn't always happen.

The same doctor talked about accommodating women's own wishes as to the type of care they would receive when considering the meaning of risk in individual cases. He went on to remark, "We don't actually sit down and say, now let's see your pregnancy and labor plans. But some come with lists, and both the younger and the more experienced [staff] people here find that very off-putting."

In our attempt to illuminate professional and personal differences in definitions of what constitutes good care, we asked two final questions about how in principle the doctors and midwives in our sample regarded the issue of women's right to choose: the issue obliquely referred to in the example just quoted, in the reactions of the young doctors who do not have a high opinion of pregnant women armed with lists. We asked, "Do you agree that pregnant women have a right to choose the kind of care they want?" In answer to this, 16 percent of the midwives said no or don't know, 29 percent of the doctors said no or don't know, and a further 24 percent of the doctors said yes, but added qualifications. Our last question concerned the controversial topic of abortion: "Do you think that women have an automatic right to abortion?" Here, 19 percent of the doctors said no, but so did 31 percent of the midwives. Surprisingly, midwives in Catholic countries were less likely to say no than those in Denmark and the United Kingdom, where abortion is legal and (relatively) easily available.

These answers also draw attention to the complex link between gender and professional perspectives. All the midwives in our sample were women; most of the obstetricians were men. This reflects real-world gender divisions. While the two professional groups seem to differ in the direction of the (female) midwives being more sensitive to the individual psychosocial and medical needs of childbearing women, this bias toward woman-centered care has to compete with what might be termed a lack of feminist awareness in much professional midwifery training. Professional ideologies are themselves to some extent part of the masculine world view, and indoctrination by them is capable of changing other social allegiances.

Chapter Eight

The Invisible Vision

The future of midwives, the future of childbirth, and the future of motherhood—all these are part of the same pattern, the same struggle.

When we speak of women, babies, and midwives, however, we speak of social groups who lack power. Considered in the political context of a male-dominated social order and a health care system controlled by professionalized medicine and influenced by commercial interests, a woman and her child and the woman who is with her when she gives birth to it are dependent on others to write their scripts for them. They come on stage when cued, speak their lines, briefly occupy the center of the stage, and then walk off again. The play is written by somebody else; somebody else has arranged and allocated the actors' parts, has arbitrated the nature of the drama, has decided how it should be carved up into separate acts. Somebody else gets the credit when the play does well and is cheered by audiences and critics; somebody else collects the royalties at the end of the day.

We have seen in this book some of the ways in which midwives and childbearing women today have their parts written for them. We have seen how the education, training, and legislation relating to midwifery have prescribed a limited role for the midwife in the care of women having babies: she is only to be the manager of normal childbearing. One might think this is enough. Not so, because it is not the midwife who defines what is normal; obstetricians do that.

We have seen how the increasing hospitalization of childbirth and the enthusiasm for technology and for intervention have encroached even further on the space occupied by the midwife, so that many now feel there is only one way out: to leave midwifery and/or the official system of care altogether (to the detriment, it must be said, of the women they leave behind them).

We have seen how the midwife is trapped by the idea of risk that is so close to the heart of the obstetrician; everywhere she looks, she is instructed to remember the possibility of death, at the same time as she knows that the risk of death is not the only important aspect of childbirth she or any of us has to confront. Childbirth is about the possibility of life; it is about renewal, hope, growth, change, optimism, a vision of the future. The midwife is a defender and a protagonist of this vision. It is this she must cherish, in alliance with the women she helps, if she is to preserve her own work in the future.

VISIONARY PRINCIPLES

In 1986, the Association of Radical Midwives (ARM) in the United Kingdom drew up a document outlining a possible future for the maternity services. It was called *The Vision*. Although ARM is a minority voice even among British midwives, the principles underlying *The Vision* emerge from, and thus provide a valuable way of summarizing, much of the material surveyed in this book.

There are eight basic principles:

1 The relationship between mother and midwife is fundamental to good midwifery care.
2 The mother herself is the central person in the process of care.
3 Midwives' skills should be fully used.
4 All childbearing women must have continuity of care.
5 Care should be community-based.
6 Women should have choice in childbirth.
7 The maternity services should be accountable to those who use them.
8 Care should cause no harm to mother and baby.

Using these principles, ARM produced a plan for a remodeled maternity service, in which midwives would be the "recognized portals of entry" into care for all pregnant women. According to the plan, 60 percent of the midwives would be community-based and would work from group practices. These midwives would care for the majority of women, who are expected to pass through childbirth without complications. They would deliver some at home and some in hospital, "according to individual circumstances and individual choice." The remaining 40 percent of midwives would be hospital-based and would work in teams with consultants, looking after women who have problems. Even in hospital, the principle of continuity of care is to be preserved through teamwork.

Midwives in the community would have direct access to specialist services, such as ultrasound, and to consultant obstetricians for advice. Decisions to transfer a woman from the community to hospital for her care would only be made by the midwife, consultant, and woman together. All midwifery training would be by direct entry. As well as clinical midwifery skills and basic anatomy and physiology, all midwifery education programs would include counseling, communication skills, psychology, sociology, epidemiology, research methods, political awareness, information about rights and disciplinary procedures, and assertiveness training.

This scheme is clearly a far cry from what happens in most places today. It is ambitious, yet vague about some critical factors—for example, about who is to determine the allocation of women between community and hospital care, and how this is to be done. Nevertheless, *The Vision* has the appeal of restoring the experience of normal childbirth to both midwives and women—and of restoring it as an area of life whose character and autonomy properly go far beyond the subject matter and jurisdiction of professionalized medicine.

Outlining alternatives to an existing system is an act of imagination. This can have the effect of making people take a new look at something overly familiar. A well-known experiment with playing cards demonstrates the way this process can work. In the experiment, people are asked to look at a set of playing cards flashed on a screen. Most of the cards are perfectly standard ones, but a few are anomalous—a red seven of clubs, for instance. When the cared are flashed quickly in front of people, the anomalous cards are "normalized"—people do not pick them out as unusual. When given longer to look at each card, however, after some hesitation, the people taking part in the experiment identify each card correctly, describing even the anomalous ones correctly.

Something similar happens when hospital midwives begin to experience home birth. The previous perception of all pregnancies and labors as fitting—or needing to fit—the old set of standard rules vanishes, and in its place childbearing women become individuals who normally behave in different ways. The rules themselves then begin to be questioned—for example, the rule about the safe length of second-stage labor or the one about depriving the laboring woman of food and drink. The end result of this process is that *facts* are relabeled as *artifacts*. The medical setting is understood to produce one kind of truth, the experience of normal birth in the community another. Unfortunately, it is sometimes true that new rules arise to replace the old; an emphasis on the normality of childbirth is no guarantee against this.

Changing childbirth and midwifery is thus, in part, an effort of the imagination. In a 1982 critique of the concept of choice in childbirth, in the journal

Birth, social psychologist Martin Richards talked about the fixed assumption that childbirth technology can only be used in the hospital:

> To a greater or lesser extent machines embody assumptions about how, when and where they should be used. For example, much obstetric equipment is designed on the assumption that it will be used in one place—say in the delivery room—rather than be transported from house to house for home deliveries. At least the earlier forms of fetal monitoring took it for granted that the mother would be in bed so that she could be attached by wires to a machine, and that her membranes would be ruptured early in labor, so that a clip could be placed on the baby's scalp. Once machines have been produced on these assumptions, the existence of the machine in its particular form becomes a reason for not changing practices—a determinant of practice. . . . As long as fetal monitoring involves attaching a mother by wires to a machine, its existence will be used as an argument against mothers moving around during labor. Characteristics of machines are not limitations imposed by the possibilities of engineering but are conceptual. They are ideas and assumptions in the minds of those who design and use machines.

Machines are designed with a certain system of social relations around birth in mind. With a different system of social relations, there will be different machines, including those that permit decentralization of care: portable sonicaids and ultrasound scanners, telephone transmission of fetal monitoring patterns, and so on.

PROFESSION: TO BE OR NOT TO BE?

We end this book with a few provocative thoughts about the status of midwifery as an occupation.

It is widely assumed that what is wrong with midwifery today is that its professional status is not as high as it ought to be—not as high as that of medicine, for example. Thus, the argument goes, to regain a central place in the control of childbirth, midwives must fight for further professionalization: tighter controls over practice, more specialized knowledge, and so on. At first sight, this argument appears sound, but it is seriously flawed. The problem is that the consequences of professionalization may run counter to the reasons for defending the profession in the first place. Midwives, in short, may become more like doctors instead of more like midwives.

For any group to turn itself into a profession, the first thing that has to happen is some form of licensing. The sociologist Raymond DeVries, who has worked extensively on the issue of the meaning for midwifery practice of licensing and regulation, identified a somewhat sinister dual purpose behind these activities in a paper in the journal *Research in the Sociology of Heath Care* in 1982. When the state and the medical profession came together in various countries in the nineteenth and early twentieth centuries to produce midwifery legislation, they both recognized midwifery work as important and tried to control it. In the years when midwifery regulation was being most actively discussed in the United Kingdom and the United States:

> Most physicians opposed the registration of midwives on the grounds that legal recognition would enhance the midwife's position, take births away from doctors and hinder the development of obstetrics. While many doctors regarded assisting in birth as a time-consuming and often messy and manual task, it was felt to be an important way of developing and maintaining a clientele. On the other hand, and for many of the same reasons, midwives were often anxious to see some type of licensing law passed, viewing such legislation as a necessary condition for survival. On the surface these positions seem consistent with the best interests of the occupations involved, but if the outcomes of midwife regulation are investigated, this assumption becomes questionable. Contrary to the beliefs of both doctors and midwives, these regulatory acts did not result in the establishment of an independent profession of midwifery, but rather placed the midwife in a position where her autonomy has steadily declined.

Here, history provides one answer to the contemporary debate about the licensing of lay midwifery in places where it is still treated as illegal. Licensing has a double message: to recognize the value of what midwives do and to limit what in the future they will be able to do. The result of licensing is most likely to be that the licensed midwife would be "forced to operate in medical settings, only after a sustained period of medically directed training." This, in turn, affects midwife-client relations and, indeed, the whole nature of midwife-attended birth.

Studies of licensed lay midwifery in the United States suggest that this is in fact what is happening. One such study was undertaken in 1982 by Rose Weitz and Deborah Sullivan in Arizona. There were only three practicing licensed midwives in the state of Arizona in 1977, although a law had been passed twenty years earlier allowing the licensing of lay midwives who met certain minimal qualification criteria. However, pressure from practicing illegal midwives in the 1970s led the state Department of Health Services to adopt new rules and regulations in 1978. The new rules required prospective midwives to show evidence of formal training in midwifery.

Weitz and Sullivan interviewed twenty-seven of the twenty-nine women licensed to practice midwifery between 1977 and 1982. All the midwives they talked to supported a nonmedical definition of childbirth: pregnancy, labor, and delivery are natural healthy events. Yet, in practice, after being licensed, these midwives increasingly took a medical risk-based approach. As they delivered more and more babies under the new system of regulation, they began to reassess their belief that childbirth is inherently normal. Their daily contact with the medical world and its particular repertoire of behavior, attitudes, and ideologies made them revise their approach. The relationship with the medical domain, itself a consequence of regulation, proved to be the critical factor. Licensing usually makes midwives directly dependent on doctors even for the right to practice; they must pass an examination administered by physicians.

Five years after the new licensing procedures were introduced in Arizona, the midwives' practices had become more similar to those of the doctors. They emphasized risk more and talked more about technology. Although they saw technology as appropriate only in an emergency, some wanted to be allowed to carry more of it routinely, so that they *could* use it in the event of possible complications. The licensed midwives' attitudes toward their clients had also changed. Despite the fact that they continued to stress women's rights to information and choice in childbirth, the midwives said that sometimes their professional expertise requires them to override their clients' wishes and decisions.

The phrase *the profession of midwifery* is to some a contradiction in terms. Although many midwives think of their occupation as a profession, and would like it to be more so, when viewed sociologically, midwifery is not a profession at all.

To be a profession, a group has to have autonomy—autonomy to set its own standards of practice for its own members. This midwifery can do to only a limited extent. Medicine lays down the ground rules for midwives to follow. A further condition required for professionalization is control over clientele. Doctors possess this; hence, much of the literature on relationships between doctors and their patients emphasizes themes of power and control and their converses, dependency and submission. Midwives do not formally exercise that kind of control over childbearing women, although they may do so informally in practice when attending women having babies. (It is sometimes the case that informal power is exercised as a reaction to the lack of formally recognized power: the relations of mothers and small children may be a parallel case.)

Behind these complex issues of midwifery and power, it may be the case that the idea of the midwife as "being with woman" has nothing whatsoever to do with the modern notion of a profession. It may be something else altogether—something much older, much more fundamental, much more challenging to the modern scientific world, obsessed as it is with the quantification of biological parameters of experience, with death and illness rates as measures of the comparative health of populations, and with the notions that to cure is better than to care, and that to tell people what is good for them is better than allowing them to stumble onto this truth for themselves.

As it is put in *The Vision* (1986), "midwives are unique in their combination of skill, sensitivity, and training, to be "with woman" through one of life's landmark experiences which has longterm effects on the individual, the family, and society as a whole. We must generate a new feeling in midwifery. We owe it to ourselves and to those we serve."

Bibliography

CHAPTER 1

Brooks, E. F. *Nurse Practitioners, Certified Nurse-Midwives and Physician Assistants: Quality, Access, Economic, and Payment Issues.* Case study for the Office of Technology Assessment. Washington, D.C.: Office of Technology Assessment, 1985.

van Daalen, R. Dutch obstetric care: home or hospital, midwife or gynaecologist? *Health Promotion* 2(3): 247–255.

Davis, E. *A Guide to Midwifery: Heart and Hands.* Sante Fe, N.M.: John Muir Publications, 1981.

Gaskin, I. M. *Spiritual Midwifery.* Summertown, Tenn.: The Book Publishing Co., 1980.

Golden, J. "Midwifery Training: The Views of Newly Qualified Midwives." Paper presented at conference, "Research and the Midwife," London, 1979.

Having a Baby in Europe. Public Health in Europe, No. 26. Copenhagen: WHO Regional Office for Europe, 1985.

Hessing-Wagner, J. *Samenhang in de zorg rond geboorte en jonge kinderen.* Rijswijk: Sociaal en Cultureel Planbureau, 1985.

Kargar, I. "The Night Shift." *Association of Radical Midwives Magazine*, no. 30 (Autumn, 1986): 16–18.

Weig, M. "An independent streak." *Nursing Times* (25 January 1984): 16–18.

CHAPTER 2

Alexander, G. A. "A Survey of Traditional Medical Practices Used for the Treatment of Malignant Tumours in an East African Population." *Social Science and Medicine* 20(1) (1985): 53–59.

Arney, W. R. *Power and the Profession of Obstetrics.* Chicago: University of Chicago Press, 1982.

Bent, E. A. "The Growth and Development of Midwifery." In *Nursing, Midwifery and Health Visiting since 1900,* edited by P. Allan and M. Jolley. London: Faber and Faber, 1982.

Chamberlain, M. *Old Wives' Tales: Their History, Remedies, and Spells.* London: Virago, 1981.

Clark, A. *Working Life of Women in the Seventeenth Century.* London: Frank Cass, 1968.

Demos, J. "Underlying Themes in the Witchcraft of Seventeenth Century New England." *American Historical Review* (1970): 1311–26

Devitt, M. "The Statistical Case for the Elimination of the Midwife: Fact Versus Prejudice 1890–1935. Part I. *Women and Health,* 4(1) (1979): 81–96, Haworth Press, Inc., 10 Alice St., Binghamton, NY 13904. Copyright © 1979.

———. "The Statistical Case for the Elimination of the Midwife: Fact Versus Prejudice 1890–1935. Part II." *Women and Health* 4(2) (1979): 169–87.

Donnison, J. *Midwives and Medical Men.* London: Heinemann, 1976.

Ehrenreich, B., & D. English. *Witches, Midwives and Nurses.* London: Writers and Readers Publishing Cooperative, 1976.

Garrigues, H. J. *A Textbook of the Science and Art of Obstetrics.* Philadelphia: Lippincott, 1902.

Grey, E. *Cottage Life in a Hertfordshire Village.* Harpenden: Harpenden and District Local Historical Society, 1977.

Hughes, M. J. *Women Healers in Medieval Life and Literature.* New York: Kings Crown Press, 1943.

Kramer, H., & H. J. Sprenger. *The Malleus Maleficarum.* New York: Dover Publications, 1971.

Leedam, E. "Traditional Birth Attendants." *International Journal of Gynecology and Obstetrics* 23(4) (1985): 249–74.

Levin, L. S., & E. L. Idler. *The Hidden Health Care System: Mediating Structures and Medicine.* Cambridge, Mass.: Ballinger, 1981.

Litoff, J. B. *American Midwives 1860 to the Present.* Westport, Conn.: Greenwood Press, 1978.

Newbold, D. "The Value of Male Nurses in Maternity Care." *Nursing Times* (17 October 1984).

Oakley, A. "Wisewoman and Medicine Man: Changes in the Management of Childbirth." In *The Rights and Wrongs of Women,* edited by J. Mitchell and A. Oakley. Harmondsworth: Penguin, 1976.

Oyebola, D. D. O. "Traditional Medicine and Its Practitioners among the Yoruba of Nigeria: A Classification." *Social Science and Medicine* 14A (1980): 23–29.

———. "The Method of Training Traditional Healers and Midwives among the Yoruba of Nigeria." *Social Science and Medicine* 14A (1980): 31–37.

Savage, W. *A Savage Enquiry.* London: Virago, 1986.
Scarpa, A. "Pre-Scientific Medicines: Their Extent and Value." *Social Science and Medicine* 15A (1981): 317–26.
Sousa, M. *Childbirth at Home.* Englewood Cliffs, N.J.: Prentice Hall, 1976.
Thomas, K. *Religion and the Decline of Magic: Studies in Popular Beliefs in Sixteenth and Seventeenth Century England.* London: Weidenfeld and Nicholson, 1971.
Versluysen, M. "Lying-in Hospitals in Eighteenth Century London." In *Women, Health and Reproduction,* edited by H. Roberts. London: Routledge and Kegan Paul, 1981.

CHAPTER 3

Brooks, E. F. *Nurse Practitioners, Certified Nurse-Midwives and Physician Assistants: Quality, Access, Economic, and Payment Issues.* Washington, D.C.: Office of Technology Assessment, 1985.
Facing the Figures: What Really Is Happening to the National Health Service? London: Radical Statistics Health Group, 1987.
Flint, C., & P. Poulengeriss. "The Know-Your-Midwife Scheme." London, 1986. Typescript.
Garcia, J., et al. "Midwives Confined? Labour ward policies and routines." Paper presented at conference, "Research and the Midwife," London, 1985.
Garcia, J., et al. "The Policy and Practice in Midwifery Study: Introduction and Methods." *Midwifery* 3 (1987): 2–9.
Garforth, S., & J. Garcia. "Admitting—A Weakness or a Strength? Routine Admission of a Woman in Labor." *Midwifery* 3 (1987): 10–24.
Having a Baby in Europe. Public Health in Europe, No. 26. Copenhagen: WHO Regional Office for Europe, 1985.
Henderson, C. "Influences and Interactions Surrounding the Midwife's Decision to Rupture the Membranes." Paper presented at conference, "Research and the Midwife," London, 1984.
Kirkham, M. "Information-Giving by Midwives During Labour." Paper presented at conference, "Research and the Midwife," London, 1981.
Klaus, M. H., et al. "Effects of Social Support During Parturition on Maternal and Infant Morbidity." *British Medical Journal* 293 (1986): 585–87.
Legislation Concerning Nursing/Midwifery Services and Education. Copenhagen: WHO Regional Office for Europe, 1981.
Methven, R. M. "The Antenatal Booking Interview: Recording an Obstetric History or Relating with a Mother-to-Be?" Paper presented at conference, "Research and the Midwife," London, 1982, pp. 63–76.
Newsom, K. "Direct Entry Method of Training Midwives in Three Countries: 1, The Netherlands." *Midwives' Chronicle and Nursing Notes* (February, 1981) 39–43.
Olds, D. L., et al. "Improving the Delivery of Prenatal Care and Outcomes of Pregnancy: A Randomized Trial of Nurse Home Visitation." *Pediatrics* 77(1) (1986): 16–28.
Perry, H. B. "Role of the Nurse-Midwife in Contemporary Maternity Care." In *Psycho-*

somatic Obstetrics and Gynecology, edited by D. D. Youngs & A. A. Enrhardt New York: Appleton-Century-Crofts, 1980.

Reid, M. E., et al. *A Comparison of the Delivery of Antenatal Care Between a Hospital and a Peripheral Clinic.* Glasgow: Social Paediatric and Obstetric Research Unit, 1984.

Robinson, S., et al. *A Study of the Role and Responsibilities of the Midwife.* London: Nursing Education and Research Unit, Department of Nursing Studies, Chelsea College, University of London, 1983.

Runnerstrom, L. "The Effectiveness of Nurse-Midwifery in a Supervised Hospital Environment." *American College of Nurse Midwives Bulletin* 14(2) (1969): 40–52.

Sampson, R. V. *The Psychology of Power.* New York: Pantheon, 1966.

Slome, C., et al. "Effectiveness of Certified Nurse-Midwives." *American Journal of Obstetrics and Gynecology* 15(1) (1976): 177–82.

Spira, N., et al. "Surveillance à domicile des grossesses pathologiques par les sages-femmes." *Journal of Gynaecology, Obstetrics, Biology and Reproduction* 10 (1981): 543–48.

White, S. M., et al. "Emergency Obstetric Surgery Performed by Nurses in Zaire." *Lancet* (12 September 1987): 612–13.

CHAPTER 4

Breen, Dana. *The Birth of a First Child.* London: Tavistock, 1975.

Chamberlain, G. V. P., & A. Oakley. "Medical and Social Factors in Postpartum Depression." *Journal of Obstetrics and Gynaecology* 1 (1981): 182–87.

Engelmann, G. J. *Labor among Primitive Peoples.* St. Louis, Mo.: J. H. Chambers, 1883.

Flint, C. *Sensitive Midwifery.* London: Heinemann, 1986.

Gaskin, I. M. *Spiritual Midwifery.* Sommertown, Tenn.: The Book Publishing Co., 1978.

Having a Baby in Europe. Public Health in Europe, No. 26. Copenhagen: WHO Regional Office for Europe, 1985.

Jordan, B. *Birth in Four Cultures: A Cross-Cultural Investigation of Childbirth in Yucatan, Holland, Sweden, and the United States.* 2nd edition. Montreal: Eden Press Women's Publications, 1980.

Mead, M., & N. Newton "Cultural Patterning of Perinatal Care." In *Childbearing—Its Social and Psychological Aspects,* edited by S. A. Richardson & A. F. Guttmacher. Baltimore: Williams & Wilkins, 1967.

Nelson, M. K. "Working Class Women, Middle Class Women and Models of Childbirth." *Social Problems* 30(3) (1983): 285–96

Oakley, A. "Obstetric Practice—Cross-Cultural Comparisons." In *Psychobiology of the Human Newborn,* edited by P. Stratton. New York: John Wiley & Sons, 1982.

Phaff, J. M. L., ed. *Perinatal Health Services in Europe: Searching for Better Childbirth* (Table 6.1, p. 83). London: Croom Helm, 1986.

CHAPTER 5

Adams, C. J. "Nurse-Midwifery Practice in the United States 1982." *American Journal of Public Health* 74(11) (1984): 1267–70.

"Appropriate Technology Following Birth." *Lancet* (13 December 1986): 1387–88.

"Appropriate Technology for Birth." *Lancet* 24 (1985): 436–37.

Appropriate Technology for Thermal Control of Newborn Babies. Geneva: World Health Organization, 1986.

Bakketeig, L. S., & P. Bergsjoe. "Birth During Transportation." *Norske-laegeforening* (1977): 923–70.

Banta, D. "Appropriate perinatal technology." Paper presented at the Joint Interregional Conference on Appropriate Technology for Birth, Fortaleza, Brazil, 1985.

Bennetts, A. B., & R. W. Lubic. "The Free-Standing Birth Centre." *Lancet* (13 February 1982): 378–80.

Campbell, R., & A. Macfarlane. *Where to Be Born? The Debate and the Evidence.* Oxford: National Perinatal Epidemiology Unit, 1987.

Dening, F. "Alternative Positions in Childbirth." *Midwives' Chronicle and Nursing Notes* (July 1982): 256–57.

Directory of Maternity and Postnatal Care Organizations. Ipswich, Suffolk: Association for Improvements in the Maternity Services, 1984. (Compiled by the Ipswich Group of AIMS.)

Eakins, P. S., & G. A. Richwald. *Free-Standing Birth Centers in California: Structure, Cost, Medical Outcome and Issues.* Berkeley, California: Department of Health Services, Maternal and Child Health Branch, 1986.

Fraser, C. M. "Selected Perinatal Procedures: Scientific Basis for Use and Psychosocial Effects: A Literature Review." *Acta Obstetrica et Gynecologica Scandinavica* Suppl. 117 (1983): entire issue.

Freeman, R. *Women and Health—The Lay Component.* Copenhagen: WHO Regional Office for Europe, 1982.

Gillett, J. "Childbirth in Pithiviers, France." *Lancet* (27 October 1979): 894–96.

Hatch, S., & I. Kickbusch, eds. *Self-Help and Health in Europe.* Copenhagen: WHO Regional Office for Europe, 1983.

Health and Disease. Milton Keynes, England: Open University, 1985.

Health and the Status of Women. Geneva: World Health Organization, 1980.

van den Heuvel, W. J. A. "The Role of the Consumer in Health Policy." *Social Science and Medicine* 14A (1980): 423–26.

Klee, L. "Home Away from Home: The Alternative Birth Center." *Social Science and Medicine* 23(1) (1986): 9–16. Copyright © 1986, Pergamon Press PLC, reprinted with permission.

Leboyer, F. *Pour une Naissance sans Violence.* Paris: Editions du Sueil, 1974.

Leedam, E. "Traditional Birth Attendants." *International Journal of Obstetrics and Gynecology* 23 (1985): 249–74.

Macfarlane, A., & M. Mugford. *Birth Counts: Statistics of Pregnancy and Childbirth.* London: HM Stationery Office, 1984.

Macintyre, S. "Myth of the Golden Age." *World Medicine* 12(18) (1977).

McKay, S., & C. S. Mahan. "Laboring Patients Need More Freedom to Move." *Contemporary Obstetrics/Gynaecology* (July 1984): 17–22.

National Perinatal Epidemiology Unit and World Health Organization. *A Classified Bibliography of Controlled Trials in Ferinatal Medicine 1940–1984*. Oxford: Oxford University Press, 1985.

Pillsbury, B. L. K. "Policy and Evaluation Perspectives on Traditional Health Practitioners in National Health Care Systems." *Social Science and Medicine* 16 (1982): 1825–34.

Post, S. "Family-Centered Maternity Care: The Canadian Picture." *Dimensions in Health Service* (June 1981): 26–31.

Praeger, M., & M. Scruggs. "Pilot Project of the Characteristics of 500 Planned Home Births." Typescript, 1982.

Rakusen, J. "Feminism and the Politics of Health." *Medicine in Society* 8(I) (1982): 17–30.

Reid, M. "Apprenticeship into Midwifery: An American Example." *Midwifery* 2 (1986): 126–34.

Reid, M. "Is There a Place for the Lay Midwife?" *Nursing Times* (25 August 1982): 1424–25.

Reid, M. "Lay Midwifery in the United States." Paper presented at conference, "Research and the Midwife," London, 1982.

Rifkin, S. B. "The Role of the Public in the Planning and Management and Evaluation of Health Activities and Programmes, Including Self Care." *Social Science and Medicine* 15A (1981): 377–86.

Romito, P. "The Humanizing of Childbirth: The Response of Medical Institutions to Women's Demand for Change." *Midwifery* 2 (1986): 135–40.

Romney, M. L. "Pre-Delivery Shaving: An Unjustified Assault?" *Journal of Obstetrics and Gynaecology*, 1 (1980): 33–35.

Romney, M. L., & H. Gordon. "Is Your Enema Really Necessary?" *British Medical Journal* 282 (1981): 1269–71.

Ruzek, S. B. *The Women's Health Movement*. New York: Praeger, 1979.

Safe Motherhood: An Information Test. Geneva: World Health Organization, 1987.

Studying Maternal Mortality in Developing Countries: Rates and Causes. Geneva: World Health Organization, 1987.

Traditional Birth Attendants. Geneva: World Health Organization, 1979.

Weitz, R. "English Midwives and the Association of Radical Midwives." *Women and Health* 12(1) (1987): 79–89.

Wright, M. "Verbal Disarmament." *New Generation* 2(1) (1983): 8–9.

CHAPTER 6

Banta, H. D., & J. R. Sanes. "Assessing the Social Impacts of Medical Technologies." *Journal of Community Health* 3(3) (1978): 245–58.

Chalmers, I. "Implications of the Current Debate on Obstetric Practice." In *The Place of Birth*, edited by S. Kitzinger & J. A. Davis. Oxford: Oxford University Press, 1978.

Chalmers, I., & M. Richards. "Intervention and Causal Inference in Obstetric Practice." In *Benefits and Hazards of the New Obstetrics*, edited by T. Chard & M. Richards. London: Spastics International Medical Publications, 1977.

Elliot, J. P., & J. F. Flaherty. "The Use of Breast Stimulation to Ripen the Cervix in Term Pregnancies." *American Journal of Obstetrics and Gynecology* (1 March 1983): 553-56.

Haire, D. "Fetal Effect of Ultrasound: A Growing Controversy." *Journal of Nurse-Midwifery* 29(4) (1984): 241-46.

Liebeskind, D., et al. "Diagnostic Ultrasound Effects on the DNA and Growth Patterns of Animal Cells." *Radiology* 131 (1979): 177-84.

Lumley, J. "The Irresistible Rise of Electronic Fetal Monitoring" (editorial). *Birth* 9(3) (1982): 150-51.

Moeller, J. et al. *Twelve Home Deliveries 1980-81.* Stoerstrom Country, Denmark: Kunstforlaget Graficus, 1982.

Nicholson, R. H., ed. *Medical Research with Children: Ethics, Law and Practice.* Oxford: Oxford University Press, 1986.

Risk Approach for Maternal and Child Health: A Selected Annotated Bibliography. Geneva: World Health Organization, 1981.

Stratmeyer, M. E. "Research in Ultrasound Bioeffects: A Public Health View." *Birth and the Family Journal* 7(2) (1980): 92-100.

Tew, M. "Place of Birth and Perinatal Mortality." *Journal of the Royal College of General Practitioners* 35 (1985): 390-94.

Thacker, S. B., & H. D. Banta. "Benefits and Risks of Episiotomy: An Interpretive Review of the English Language Literature." *Obstetrical and Gynecological Survey* 38(6) (1983): 322-38.

CHAPTER 7

Baruffi, G., et al. "Patterns of Obstetric Procedures Use in Maternity Care." *Obstetrics and Gynecology* 64(4) (1984): 493-98.

Bergsjoe, P., et al. "Differences in the Reported Frequencies of Some Obstetrical Interventions in Europe." *British Journal of Obstetrics and Gynaecology* 90 (1983): 628-32.

Macintyre, S. *The Attitudes of Obstetricians and Midwives—A Neglected Area of Study.* London: Forum on Maternity and the Newborn, Royal Society of Medicine, 1984.

McClain, C. S. "Perceived Risk and Choice of Childbirth Service." *Social Science and Medicine* 17(23) (1983): 1857-65.

Zambrana, R. E., et al. "Gender and Level of Training Differences in Obstetricians, Attitudes Towards Patients in Childbirth." *Women and Health* 12(1) (1987): 5-24.

CHAPTER 8

DeVries, R. G. "Midwifery and the Problem of Licensure." *Research in the Sociology of Health Care* 2 (1982): 77-129, JAI Press, Inc. Greenwich, Conn., and London, England.

Kuhn, T. S. *The Structure of Scientific Revolutions,* 2nd ed. Chicago: University of Chicago Press, 1970.

Richards, M. P. M. "The Trouble with 'Choice' in Childbirth." *Birth* 9(4) (1982): 253-59.

Rothman, B. K. "Childbirth Management and Medical Monopoly: Midwifery as (Almost) a Profession." *Journal of Nurse-Midwifery* 29(5) (1984): 300–306.

The Vision: Proposals for the Future of the Maternity Services. Manchester, England: Association of Radical Midwives, 1986.

Weitz, R., & D. A. Sullivan. *Licensed Lay Midwifery and the Medical Model of Childbirth.* Typescript. Arizona State University (n.d.).

Midwifery and WHO: A Content Analysis of Midwifery in WHO Publications from 1952 to 1983

Susanne Houd

In 1952, an expert committee on maternity care produced a report containing the first mention of midwives by the World Health Organization (WHO) (1). The report included a direct recommendation concerning midwifery, as follows:

> The expert committee on maternity care recommends to WHO that a joint expert committee composed of members of the expert advisory panels on nursing and on maternal and child health be convened at the appropriate time to give further consideration to the training of midwifery personnel at all levels. This committee should include midwife teachers among its members. It is hoped that the proposed committee will consider midwifery training requirements for the areas where maternity care is more highly developed as well as for those in which it is less well-developed. It is suggested that before the convening of such a joint committee, necessary information regarding the present patterns of maternity services and the training of personnel be collected from various countries.

The report further recommended the need to recognize "the untrained or partially untrained indigenous midwife" so as to make use of her services. It was regarded as desirable that training of these personnel should be designed to meet the needs of the country concerned. The committee also recommended that training concerning both physical and mental aspects of health should be integrated into the existing curriculum of health workers in maternity care. In this way, the health worker would get "adequate knowledge of personality structure and development," which should amount to a "broad understanding of human behaviour and should not consist of a formal course in psychiatry."

Although the report offered no specific definition of the term *midwife,* it did mention midwives several times. In antenatal care, the midwife and the physician should "share the care and supplement each other." When the birth takes place in the hospital, the physician is ultimately responsible for it, but the midwife is an important part of the team. When the delivery takes place at home, the birth is clearly the midwife's responsibility and the doctor may be there only at the midwife's invitation. In portpartum care, the midwife is an important member of the team and works closely with the health nurse. The midwife is responsible for postpartum care until the tenth day after birth. She is considered an important support to the breastfeeding mother, whether the woman is at home or in the hospital.

This report gave no concrete description of the content of the midwife's work except in prenatal care. Here, it advised her to work closely with the physician in pregnancy and birth, supplementing and assisting the physician's work. The committee clearly recognized that normal cases are the responsibility of midwives. In hospital delivery, the report advised midwives to be nurse-midwives, so that they would work closely with nurses "well-trained in obstetrics" and under physicians "skilled in obstetrics." At domiciliary deliveries, she was to be alone but backed up by a physician or flying squad consisting of an obstetrician, a trained midwife, and, if necessary, an anesthesiologist supplied with equipment for blood transfusion, resuscitation, or other procedures.

The 1952 report did not mention postgraduate training or research as options for midwives. It did, however, recommend that midwives working in hospitals and midwives and doctors involved in teaching should have some public health knowledge. At the time this report was written, there were a shortage of hospital beds and a strong tradition of home delivery in many industrialized countries. The committee realized that the proportion of home to hospital deliveries varied from country to country and was influenced by a number of factors. It declared that women with abnormal pregnancies should be delivered in hospital, but there was a diversity of opinion among committee members as to whether hospital or domiciliary delivery should be encouraged for normal pregnancies. The safety of home deliveries was considered to depend on the suitability of the home situation, access to hospital facilities, the availability of a flying squad, and on other factors, such as the availability of midwives and/or nurses and physicians adequately trained in obstetric care. Further, the committee thought it to be the case that, "given the above favourable circumstances, home delivery offers a high degree of safety and presents several advantages from an emotional and psychological viewpoint." The committee recognized that it was more difficult to satisfy the emotional and psychological needs of the mother in the hospital. It also recommended that maternity hospital rather than a general hospital was the best option for deliveries that must take place in hospital.

This report generally acknowledged the importance of psychological factors in pregnancy and delivery. As an illustration of this, the committee compared the ease with which many women in Eastern countries were able to deliver themselves with the difficulties that women in Western countries sometimes experience. The committee felt that these complications were very often due to psychological factors. The hospital environment sometimes contributed to long labor by depriving these women of the moral support they would have received if they had delivered at home.

In its conclusion, the committee recognized that no general plan could be imposed on all countries and warned that "in certain situations the development of maternity care in the economically more developed countries has not always proceeded on the soundest lines."

The committee on maternity care that made the 1952 report consisted of nine doctors, one nursing supervisor, and no midwives.

A survey of recent legislation on midwives was carried out in 1954 (2). The introduction stated that "it might not be out of place to draw the attention of the reader to certain historical facts that illustrate the development the profession has undergone and its present importance in different countries of the world. Until the beginning of this century, the delivery of women in childbirth had been the almost exclusive preserve of midwives, the medical profession offering little or no competition."

The rapid progress of medicine during the nineteenth century enabled physicians to outdistance midwives in obstetrical technique and thus to engage in larger numbers in the practice of midwifery. About the same time, the nurse began to receive public recognition owing to the activities of Florence Nightingale, but the public still did not become midwife-conscious. It persisted in considering motherhood and its problems as a matter of essentially private concern, and it has been stated that, even as late as the beginning of the present century, in the United Kingdom "in labour the doctor was called only in a grave emergency when the efforts of the midwife, in those days untrained and unregistered, had failed to effect delivery." The first Midwives Act was not, in fact, enacted in England and Wales until 1902. These remarks are not, however, of general application, for in certain European countries the public authorities had already been exercising control over midwives for more than a hundred years; legislation governing the registration and control of midwives was adopted in Austria, Norway, and Sweden in 1801, in France in 1803, in Belgium in 1818, and in Russia, the Netherlands, and Prussia in 1865.

The present situation may be summed up as follows: in countries where there is a shortage of physicians and of auxiliary medical workers, most women are still delivered by untrained midwives, whereas in countries that have well-developed public health services, a growing proportion of women (in the United States, almost all women) are delivered by physicians, midwives playing a less important part but providing nursing care before and after childbirth. There are, however, countries with well-developed public health services where this is not so. In Sweden, almost all normal deliveries, whether domiciliary or institutional, are conducted by midwives. In France and in England and Wales also, a large proportion of women are delivered by midwives.

Thirty countries answered a questionnaire, which provided data for the 1954 report; the result is a highly complex picture of the midwifery situation. In some countries, midwifery training was available only to nurses and maternity nurses in courses lasting from six to twenty-four months. Other countries had direct-entry midwifery education in courses lasting from six months to three years. Public authorities supervised all schools, whether private or government-run. Most countries included a probationary period of one to six months at the beginning of the education period, after which unsuitable students could be dismissed. Only women could become midwives.

Many countries required midwives to attend refresher courses and to pass an examination at the end of the course. In this respect, midwives differed from other medical and auxiliary medical personnel. In some countries, women can obtain a maternity nursing education either on its own or in addition to nursing training. A maternity nurse specifically cares for the woman after her delivery only.

The laws of certain countries defined the terms *midwife* and *practice of midwifery*. A midwife could be registered or licensed in two ways: either she registered once for life, or she had to renew her registration periodically. In almost all countries, only midwives could practice midwifery, except in countries where there was a shortage of midwives. The central health authorities in the British Commonwealth nations delegated all power to make decisions concerning midwives to midwives' boards. The boards handled training, approval of training schools, conditions of registration, and regulation and supervision of practice. Health officials, medical practitioners and representatives of hospitals were members, but six out of sixteen places had to be filled by midwives.

The 1954 report attempted the difficult task of describing the care given by midwives. Their work in most countries consisted of looking after women during pregnancy—only one country opposed the midwives' caring for the pregnant woman—attending the birth, and caring for the mother and child from ten days to three years after the birth. Some countries did not allow the midwife to use drugs or instruments. In most countries, the midwife could provide care only for normal pregnancies and deliveries. However, in one country, the midwife had a duty to take care of any woman in connection with childbirth, and the presence of the midwife was the right of every woman. The midwife was recognized everywhere as a completely independent practitioner.

English, Welsh, and German laws on professional regulations meant that midwives were doubly circumscribed. In the first place, they were subject to the laws of the country defining their practice. In addition, if they worked in institutions, midwives were required to conform to its rules. The report said, "Midwives in institutional practice are subject to the regulations of the establishment in which they are employed—very often under the direct supervision of a physician. In these circumstances she is not necessarily working on her own as she is in domiciliary practice, the regulations relating to which are more precise." As a point of interest, a few countries also outlined rules on professional ethics.

The rules of most countries detailed the things midwives were not allowed to do. A number of laws were concerned with how to avoid puerperal fever and when to make an internal examination. Most countries forbade midwives to use anesthetics. Some countries allowed interventions, such as rupturing the membranes, "in certain circumstances." Some interventions were only allowed when "life is endangered." The rule of all countries allowed the midwife in life-endangering situations to do whatever she thought necessary.

The circumstances that required the presence of a physician varied from country to country. In a more developed country, relatively minor events, such as vaginal bleeding, including "staining," required a doctor's attendance, whereas developing countries provided for calling the doctor later for conditions such as a clear *placenta praevia*. Although rules differed, it would generally be true to say that the more developed the country, the earlier the physician was called in. Interestingly enough, place of birth was discussed hardly at all. The midwife usually worked in the home of the pregnant woman, although sometimes she took the woman into her own home for delivery. Most laws prohibited the latter, except when specifically permitted by the health authorities.

The 1954 survey concluded: "Provisions relating to the period and nature of midwifery training vary considerably from country to country. There is a very marked tendency in countries with well-organized health services to coordinate the training of midwives with that of the nurses." The study also showed that certain countries had been able only gradually to restrict the practice of midwifery to qualified midwives; midwives who had not yet received the prescribed training had been allowed to continue to practice in areas where there were "insufficient persons."

Finally, the survey demonstrated the number and detail of laws governing midwives. It revealed how little influence midwives themselves have on the rules that control their work. The more developed the country, the fewer the rights of the midwives. The composition of the group that made the survey was not given.

The first report specifically on midwifery training was published in 1955 (3). This report addressed itself especially to those areas where maternity care services were less well developed and where auxiliary midwifery personnel were required. The report said:

Technical assistance is essential, but without an understanding of cultural backgrounds, its application is less effective. A positive approach when interpreting these factors of custom and culture will give the best opportunities to obtain progressive changes. Some customs will be found to be definitely valuable, others will have no recognized harmful effects, while a number will be considered as harmful and undesirable. Respect for the traditional beliefs that are harmless and the full utilization of those that are valuable will give the best opportunities for gaining the confidence of the mother and family.

Although this statement gave some recognition to the value of some traditional practices, it did not say, "We can learn from traditional birth attendants." The report placed the traditional birth attendant (TBA) at the bottom of the "knowledge hierarchy" of different types of midwife. Above her came the auxiliary midwife (a TBA with some training but still possibly illiterate), and in the third and top group was the fully trained midwife. The report acknowledged the social impact and importance of the TBA's knowledge of families, customs, and so forth. The committee also thought that the basic educational background of nurses and midwives should be the same. It did not actually suggest that midwives should first be nurses but did suggest that midwifery and nursing students should share some training. This philosophy also formed the committee's recommendations for training facilities and teaching personnel, although it realized the need for more and better midwifery teachers, manuals, and books. The committee suggested that WHO find ways of helping with this.

The committee responsible for the 1955 report placed the midwife in a central position in maternity care. Finally, it concluded that maternity services were undeveloped in most of the world, and went on to say that "this regrettable deficiency is essentially due to a great shortage of medical, trained midwifery and other health personnel. The TBA and auxiliary are being used to help this deficiency." Local needs were to govern the development of programs, with both practicing and training personnel acting as a team. The committee also recommended that WHO itself should support regional conferences "which will evaluate the expanding training and use of midwives in relation to maternity care programmes." Research and studies of midwifery by WHO were proposed for increasing the relevance of training programs.

The 1955 report committee consisted of eight doctors and/or public health physicians, four nurses, one nurse-midwife, and one midwife antenatal teacher.

In spite of the 1955 recommendations, a nine-year gap followed publication of the report before any further publications on midwifery emerged either from the Regional Office for Europe or from WHO headquarters. Then, in 1964, a conference was held in Moscow to examine the role of the midwife in maternity care, evaluate her contribution to the development of health care programs, and decide what kind of training she must eventually have so as to participate fully in protecting the health of the family (4). Thirty-nine people from seventeen countries participated. Of these, ten were midwives. Some countries sent two midwives, and other countries sent none. Observers, consultants, and advisers and WHO staff provided the group with three additional midwives.

Some of the main issues of this conference were the following.

1 *Place of birth.* The group pointed out that the Netherlands offered an example of home birth, but one that was hard to imitate. It noted the trend toward hospital delivery and quoted the philosophy that no birth can be called normal until it is over. Studies on the place of birth recommended.

2 *The midwife and the hospital.* In a hospital delivery, the midwife was described as forming part of the team as opposed to playing an independent role in home deliveries. The report said that midwives working in hospitals and those caring for women delivered at home had little understanding of one another and worked together poorly, if at all.

3 *The definition of a midwife as a person specializing in the care of the pregnant, birthing, and postpartum woman and the newborn.* She gave care in three different areas: prevention, health education, and detection of abnormalities. The last included the transfer of the woman and child to medical assistance and, in the absence of medical help, the ability to give emergency care. Nowhere did the word *normal* limit the extent of the midwife's work. All pregnant women passed through her hands. She screened them and thus held primary responsibility for their care. Further, the midwife had an important role as a contact person for women who were providing lay health care for their families. She was seen as the general health educator for the family as well as the natural educator and counselor on sexual matters and gynecological problems.

The underlying message of the report's recommendations, especially those on training, advised midwives to work only within an area defined by WHO and to work within these limits as a team member and not as an independent practitioner. The midwife was to stay out of decision making and politics. In addition, the report recommended locating midwifery schools in hospitals, and, although teaching and administration were mentioned as options for midwives, attending home deliveries was not. The report clearly anticipated a future in which all midwives would work in hospitals.

In 1965, a WHO expert committee reported on midwives and maternity care (5). Midwives filled five of the thirteen places in the group. The committee planned to "review the work of the midwife and to define her contribution to maternity care in the light of development and changes that have occurred during the last decade. The discussion will cover as many geographical areas as possible and consider the work of traditional birth attendants as well as that of midwives and auxiliary midwives."

This committee emphasized a major change that had occurred since the last WHO report on maternity care and midwifery training: "that in certain countries almost 100% of the mothers have their babies in hospitals, and nearly everywhere there has been an increase in hospital facilities, especially in urban areas, which has resulted in improved safety for mother and child at the time of delivery."

Mothers were said to be going home from the hospital earlier, partly because of a shortage of beds and partly because of a change in attitudes toward postnatal care. Thus, there was a division of responsibilities among midwives, in which domiciliary midwives mainly handled antenatal and postnatal care, while hospital midwives dealt with deliveries. This division of responsibility made continuity of care increasingly difficult to achieve.

Another important development was the increasing interest in midwives shown by the medical profession. As a result, midwives worked more closely with doctors, and the crowd of health professionals around the mother swelled to include the midwife along with the family doctor, pediatrician, public health nurse, health visitor, maternity nurse, and physiotherapist. A shortage of midwives in hospitals meant that auxiliary staff untrained in midwifery also took care of delivering mothers. At the same time, new responsibilities were expanding the midwives' work area. These included family planning, more work during pregnancy and the postpartum period, and more involvement in cancer detection. The committee began to acknowledge the need for midwives to conduct research, although it did not specify how this was to come about. The midwife's functions were specified: she worked completely independently throughout pregnancy, birth, and the postpartum period. Other professionals were not mentioned except in pathological cases and when the baby became the responsibility of the health visitor ten days after the birth.

The 1965 report revealed some confusion about the midwife's actual role. According to the WHO definition, she was an independent practitioner with absolute authority to decide when to refer, no matter where she practiced. Other parts of the report emphasized that, in opposition to earlier practice, she was a team member, unable to provide continuity of care in most places. The report clearly endorsed the midwife's role as health educator, however, because she could "assist at a time when her help is appreciated, she is welcomed into the homes of people in every kind of community, and therefore she can educate." She could perform this essential function because she was well known locally, and when both the midwife and the place of birth were unfamiliar, this function was lost. The report recognized the importance of domiciliary experience for all midwives.

Must midwives first be nurses? The committee thought not, mostly because of expense.

So far as TBAs were concerned, the committee thought they performed a useful role in areas where health services were not sufficiently developed. Legislation had failed to eliminate them, because families and mothers wanted their services. Since they could not eradicate TBAs, both WHO and UNICEF recommended some supervision and training for them.

An interesting part of the report dealt with the elements of successful teamwork. The midwife was seen as forming a crucial link between the team and the family, and she was said to be the person to judge whether any other team member was needed. This statement seems to be in contrast with teamwork strategies. Considerations of seniority or hierarchy were discouraged in the team. These recommendations made clear, for the first time, the right of the midwife to be involved in policy making, whether at the international, national, or local level. The report also encouraged the midwife to conduct research and, to facilitate this, "courses on research methodology might be included in postgraduate training for midwives participating in this work."

After reviewing changing patterns of maternity care, the committee concluded that the midwife's role was a permanent and essential part of that care all over the world, both in developing and developed countries. Although the expansion of the midwife's responsibilities into family planning and cancer detection was a clear recognition of her value, the committee was concerned that this might jeopardize her crucial work in maternal and child health care. Many of the report's recommendations stemmed from a desire to protect this basic midwifery function. Thus, there are recommendations that attest to the midwife's position as the person primarily responsible for maternity care. A new aspect of the efficient use of midwives was a suggestion that they assist in cases where there was a shortage of medical staff!

In 1974, the Regional Office issued a report evaluating the maternal and child health services in certain countries of the European Region (6). The report examined the content of maternal and child health services, with the aim of establishing which ones were necessary. In the light of this concern, it is rather extraordinary that the report makes no mention whatsoever of midwives. Maternal and child health were seen as a part of family health, and family health in turn was viewed as part of community health. In this particular construction, the midwife disappeared altogether. Yet, at the same time, the 1974 report introduces two new ideas with regard to maternal and child health, which have since become more and more important in their implications for the status and work of midwives. These are, first, the recognition of the importance of the users of the services in the development and evaluation of health care and, second, the risk approach in maternal and child health care. The committee that produced this report consisted of twelve physicians and one nurse-midwife.

In the same year, 1974, WHO headquarters published a report on community health nursing (7). This publication also stressed the view of maternal and child health as an integral part of family health care: "It is logical, therefore, to consider the health needs and problems of the family as a whole, and to deal with individual health problems within the framework of a comprehensive family health programme." This new formulation of family health resulted in a shift in thinking: the midwife was no longer to occupy her accustomed place as the central person in maternal health; instead, she was to act only as a member of a team of community nursing services. The consequence of this was the disappearance of midwives (at least semantically) into the ranks of nurses. For the first time, we find in a WHO publication the statement (which was to become more and more frequent in subsequent publications) that "midwifery is not mentioned specifically in discussions of nursing services, but is considered to be implicit throughout." Midwifery had been relegated to a footnote.

Again, in the same year (1974), the Regional Office held its first liaison meeting with nursing and midwifery associations (8). The purposes of this meeting were "to consider the basic concepts which underlie the effective development of nursing/ midwifery services and to suggest ways in which the Regional Office could contribute to their application'' and ''to identify nursing functions more clearly and concurrently, and the major problems and constraints confronting the profession in discharging them.'' Another purpose of the meeting was to suggest ways of improving communication among nongovernmental organizations and between these organizations and the Regional Office. Representatives from organizations all over Europe participated, including thirteen nurses, three doctors, and two midwives. This list of participants reflected the lesser importance given to midwifery at the meeting. A footnote in the report stated that ''the majority of midwives in the world are not nurses; in many of the countries of Europe midwifery is recognized as a separate profession.'' A representative of the International Confederation of Midwifery, present at the meeting, regretted that WHO's consistent use of the word *nurse* seemed to exclude midwifery from the remit of the meeting and from the text of the position paper. Despite the fact that several recommendations and comments in the report did clearly relate to midwives and midwifery, these were extremely limited.

In 1976, the WHO headquarters' committee on maternal and child health published its sixth report (9). The committee had decided to concentrate on the developing countries. Consequently, midwives were mentioned only as TBAs, who were regarded as suitable targets for training. The term *primary health care workers* appeared often in this report; it may have been intended sometimes to include midwives, but this was never made explicit. The members of the committee included nineteen doctors, one professor of public health, and one nurse.

In 1976, the second liaison meeting with nursing and midwifery associations took place in the European Region (10). Eleven nurses, three midwives, three representatives of health authorities, and two doctors participated. The meeting's purposes were the same as those of the first liaison meeting, and again one finds a telling footnote on the first page of the report: ''The term 'nursing' in this document is used in the generic sense and, where appropriate, is indicative of midwifery.''

At this meeting, the medium-term program of the Regional Office was presented. The major problem to be discussed was ''confusion as to the real nature of nursing and its place within overall health services.'' The group emphasized that nursing and midwifery are disciplines in their own rights and in no way could, or should, be classified or developed as paramedical professions. Although the group recognized severe problems in the functioning of the primary health team, the role of both nurses and midwives as team members was not questioned. A clear need was recognized for closer communication among all kinds of nongovernmental organizations and between Member States and WHO; mention was made of the need to encourage further meetings in which more midwives might participate.

The third liaison meeting with nursing and midwifery organizations was held in 1978, again arranged by the Nursing Unit in the Regional Office (11). Participants in this meeting included twelve nurses, three midwives, four doctors, and two others from public services. In retrospect, the group members felt that the first two meetings had been overly concerned with the WHO medium-term program. The usual footnote on midwifery appeared on the first page of the report. Of the nine summary recommendations, eight made no mention of midwifery. The ninth recommendation ''stressed the need for the revision of legislation which restricted nurses/midwives from practising as autonomous and accountable professionals.'' Included in the report was a statement from the International Confederation of Midwifery, giving a good general picture of the midwife's situation, although containing the erroneous statement that "most countries have full nursing training as a basis for midwifery" (at the time, half of Europe's midwives were still direct-entry midwives). The Nordic Midwives Association, attending for the first time, also made a statement. This association discussed how midwives from smaller countries could join together and eventually, through legislation, make if possible to work in each other's countries.

In 1980, a publication was issued on the continuing education of health personnel and its evaluation (12). This report said that continuing education programs were essential for nurses and midwives. Throughout the report, however, nurses and midwives were taken together, thus ignoring the reality that continuing education is far more difficult for midwives to secure than for nurses. By 1979, the need for continuing education for nurses was widely accepted—as, indeed, was their role in research. The continuing education of midwives and their role in research were, by contrast, scarcely recognized, and opportunities were very few and far between. Because of this disparity between nurses and midwives, the report's recommendations were much more relevant for midwives than for nurses.

The fourth liaison meeting of nursing and midwife organizations was arranged by the Regional Office in 1980 (13). Ten nurses, three midwives, two doctors, and five others participated. Previous concerns, including the development of the WHO medium-term program and the strengthening of communication both among other organizations and between WHO and Member States, was discussed. The standard footnote on midwives reappeared. One research study carried out by a Swedish midwife was reported. The International Confederation of Midwifery statements were mostly repetitions of those made at the third meeting, but there was a new emphasis on the lack of opportunities for postgraduate midwifery training. The Nordic Midwives Association reported that a few midwives had begun research projects, and that the association would disseminate the results of these through journals, which would in turn stimulate more midwives to conduct research.

In 1981, the Regional Office published a report on legislation concerning nursing and midwifery services and education (14). Because nursing and midwifery are two separate disciplines that must be treated with separate legislation at national and local levels, it was therefore necessary in this report to discuss nursing and midwifery separately. In other words, when dealing with legislation, midwifery cannot be relegated to a footnote. For example, the report commented, "The bibliography on midwifery and particularly on midwifery legislation is rather poor."

Generally, the legislation directed midwives to attend only normal women expecting normal birth, but in some countries they held the main responsibility for all cases, including family planning. In many countries, midwives also did preventive work. They were allowed to provide emergency care in almost all countries. The legislation in different countries either permitted or forbade midwives to carry out specific procedures, such as episiotomy and vacuum extraction. Legislation in some countries also covered ethical aspects of practice, particularly with regard to the obligation of providing a midwife to attend a woman on request. This document covered twenty-four countries, some quite extensively, and is a valuable report that recognizes the difference between nursing and midwifery, even in countries where midwifery is a postgraduate course on top of a basic nursing education.

The fifth nursing/midwifery liaison meeting was held in 1983 (15). Participants included ten nurses, three midwives, and eight others. One of the participating midwives was a full-time midwifery consultant for the Regional Office. There was much more focus on midwifery issues than in earlier liaison meetings. Although the usual footnote still appeared on page one, several comments directly concern midwives. There seemed to be a clearer understanding that midwives and nurses can have different problems.

During the meeting, the midwifery consultant from the Regional Office reported on the study carried out there on alternative perinatal services in Europe, North America, and Canada (16). The midwifery consultant participated in this study, and it was emphasized at the liaison meeting that more research into midwifery (and by midwives) needs to be done.

Twenty-one Member States sponsored a resolution at the Thirty-Sixth World Health Assembly in 1983 on the role of nursing/midwifery personnel. This was the first time that an official public definition of these two basic health professions had been made; it finally reflected WHO's acceptance of the importance cf nursing and midwifery.

This content analysis of WHO publications reveals some rather clear trends. The first is increasing definition of the individual, independent practicing midwife as a team member. The first reports, made early in the life of the organization, fully accepted the independence of the midwife. However, as time passed and more reports were made, she became a cog in the health team wheel.

The second general trend is the disappearance of the basic psychosocial and cultural role of the midwife. Over time, what has been substituted for this is her membership of a technical team. Related to this trend is the acceptance and promotion of the value of domiciliary delivery in the early publications and the more recent, equally enthusiastic acceptance and promotion of hospital delivery.

The third major trend is the gradual overall disappearance of the midwife from WHO publications. While in the 1950s entire reports were devoted to her work, by the mid-1960s she had become a series of footnotes in nursing reports. She did, however, retain separate recognition in one way: through legislation. Since in the real world midwives are a separate profession with separate training and rules of practice, there exists a separate body of legislation that must be dealt with when studying nursing and midwifery legislation.

As a basic primary health care worker, albeit one with low status, the midwife has been shunted back and forth within WHO according to the needs of higher status health workers. With the most recent emphasis on primary health care and primary health care workers, the midwife is slowly beginning to reemerge as an essential member of the primary health care team. In a small but significant way, the most recent reports have begun to acknowledge her role in research and teaching, as well as in giving essential primary health care to childbearing women and their families.

REFERENCES

1. *Maternity Care: First Report of the Expert Committee on Maternity Care.* WHO Technical Report Series, No. 51. Geneva: World Health Organization, 1952.
2. *Midwives, a Survey of Recent Legislation.* Geneva: World Health Organization, 1954.

3. *Midwifery Training: First Report of the Expert Committee on Maternity Care.* WHO Technical Report Series, No. 93. Geneva: World Health Organization, 1955.

4. *Midwifery Education and Services: Report on a Conference.* Copenhagen: WHO Regional Office for Europe, 1965.

5. *The Midwife in Maternity Care: Report on a WHO Expert Committee.* Geneva: World Health Organization, 1965.

6. *Evaluation of MCH Services in Certain Countries of the European Region.* Copenhagen: WHO Regional Office for Europe, 1974.

7. *Community Health Nursing: Report of a WHO Expert Committee.* WHO Technical Report Series, No. 558. Geneva: World Health Organization, 1974.

8. *Report on First Liaison Meeting with Nursing/Midwifery Association on WHO's European Nursing/Midwifery Programme.* Copenhagen: WHO Regional Office for Europe, 1974.

9. *New Trends and Approaches in the Delivery of Maternal and Child Care in Health Services: Sixth Report of the WHO Expert Committee on Maternal and Child Health.* WHO Technical Report Series, No. 600. Geneva: World Health Organization, 1975.

10. *Report on Second Liaison Meeting with Nursing/Midwifery Association on WHO's European Nursing/Midwifery Programme.* Copenhagen: WHO Regional Office for Europe, 1976.

11. *Report on Third Liaison Meeting with Nursing/Midwifery Association on WHO's European Nursing/Midwifery Programme.* Copenhagen: WHO Regional Office for Europe, 1978.

12. *Continuing Education of Health Personnel and Its Evaluation.* Copenhagen: WHO Regional Office for Europe, 1980.

13. *Report on Fourth Liaison Meeting with Nursing/Midwifery Association on WHO's European Nursing/Midwifery Programme.* Copenhagen: WHO Regional Office for Europe, 1980.

14. *Legislation Concerning Nursing and Midwifery Services and Education.* Copenhagen: WHO Regional Office for Europe, 1981.

15. *Report on Fifth Liaison Meeting with Nursing/Midwifery Association on WHO's European Nursing/Midwifery Programme.* Copenhagen: WHO Regional Office for Europe, 1983.

16. *Having a Baby in Europe.* Public Health in Europe 26. Copenhagen: WHO Regional Office for Europe, 1985, 37–55.

The Role of the Midwife in Perinatal Technology in Kazakhstan, U.S.S.R.

WHO Collaborating Centre for Primary Health Care Institute of Regional Pathology, Alma-Ata, U.S.S.R.

Glossary

Midwife

A medical officer (with secondary education) who provides obstetrical, gynecological, and curative and preventive care.

Perinatal technology

A complexity of curative and preventive measures provided to pregnant women and women in labor.

Feldsher-midwifery unit

A curative and preventive establishment where primary medical care is provided to rural population groups by middle-level health personnel.

This document was provided by the Alma-Ata Collaborating Centre for Primary Health Care in response to a WHO initiative requesting collaboration with a survey of midwifery work. The center was asked to administer the risk questionnaire referred to in Chapter 7, and apparently did so.

LOCATIONS, MATERIALS, AND METHODS
OF INVESTIGATION

Objects

This investigation was carried out at obstetrical care establishments in Alma-Ata as well as in the region of Alma-Ata, Kazakhstan S.S.R.

The Kazakh S.S.R. is situated in the Southwest of the Asian part of the U.S.S.R. and covers a vast area, from the southern foothills of the Urals to the mountains of Tien-Shan; from the Caspian Sea to the plains of western Siberia. Kazakhstan is the second largest (2.7 million km^2) of the Union of Republics. The population of the Kazakh S.S.R. (16 million) is the fourth largest in the U.S.S.R. The Kazakhs are one of the five largest socialist groups in the U.S.S.R. Over half the population of Kazakhstan live in towns (there are 82 cities and 194 urban settlements in the republic). The region of Alma-Ata is an administrative area in the Southeast of the Kazakh S.S.R. with a population of 848,000 (excluding Alma-Ata): the urban population within it comprises 166,000 inhabitants.

Alma-Ata is the capital of the Kazakh S.S.R. It is situated in the Southeast of the republic, north of Tien-Shan Mountain, at the foothills of the northern slopes of the Zailisski Alatau Mountains. It is located at a height of 600–900 m above sea level in the valleys of the rivers Bolshaya, Alma-Atinka, and Malaya Alma-Atinka. Alma-Ata, with its population of one million, is one of the largest cities in the country.

Methods and Materials

Historical records. In the course of the investigation, historical documents were used relating to medical care provision for the women of Kazakhstan during pregnancy, childbirth, and the postnatal period.

Legal records. For the description of the rights and duties of midwives and the organization of obstetric care, legislative documents and methodological instructions of the U.S.S.R. and the Kazakh S.S.R. Ministry of Public Health were consulted.

Questionnaires and interviews. As part of the historical research, Kazakh women aged sixty to seventy years and over (natives of the main territories and known, in the past, as local traditional midwives) were questioned using a special questionnaire. The data obtained were compared with those found in traditional Kazakh medical literature. This stage of the research was carried out by members of the Medical History Department of the Research Institute of Regional Pathology of the Kazakh S.S.R. Ministry of Public Health.

The sample consisted of seventy people: 31 percent physicians, 63 percent midwives, and 6 percent nurses. Ninety-six percent of the people questioned were women. Their age distribution was as follows: 27 percent were aged twenty to twenty-nine years, 44 percent were aged thirty to thirty-nine years, 18 percent were aged forty to forty-nine years, and 11 percent were aged fifty years and over. Twenty-three percent had up to thirty-five years of service, 30 percent up to ten years, and 24 percent up to twenty years. Nineteen percent of all the respondents were rural inhabitants.

In addition to the scheme suggested by the WHO Regional Office for Europe, twenty cases of midwives attending women in childbirth were observed.

TRADITIONAL OBSTETRIC CARE IN KAZAKHSTAN

In recent years, a number of studies of traditional obstetric care before the revolution in Kazakhstan have been published. According to these sources, the main features of traditional obstetric care were as follows.

- The attendant for women in labor was the *kyndik-sheshe* (literally "mother ligating the umbilical cord"). She was competent and skillful in midwifery. The methods of midwifery differed between provinces and *yuezds*, depending on local customs and traditions.
- During labor, the women were allowed to walk, supported by their attendants. The custom of upright delivery was widespread. Sometimes, women would deliver their babies while on their knees, with the body leaning forward and supported by the attendants. A squatting position was also very common.
- The attendants placed the woman in labor in the appropriate position and would stand behind her, slowly tightening a wide bandage over the anterior abdominal wall of the expectant mother.
- In cases of difficult labor, the procedure would be as follows: a person (male or female) would stand behind the women in labor, placing one knee against her lower back and both arms around the upper part of her abdomen, and would apply pressure on her uterus.
- In uterine inertia as well as in cases of prolonged pregnancy, psychological methods, such a soothing, reassuring words, were applied, and walking and other forms of exercise were recommended. According to one authority, the percentage of rapid birth (less than twenty-four hours) was 71, and difficult labor only happened in 18 percent of cases.
- Following delivery of an infant, the midwife ligated the umbilical cord with clean tape or with a *taramys* (made from the tendon of a sheep). The umbilical cord was ligated about a *vershok* and a half (6.6 cm) from the infant's body. The infant was then washed with warm water containing ashes and fat. If the infant did not cry or breathe, emetic motions were induced by irritating the throat with a goose feather. Vomiting was also induced to empty the stomach contents of amniotic fluid (which the newborn may have swallowed during the delivery process).
- The placenta was removed by application of pressure. However, if the placenta was not expelled, the woman was made to blow air forcefully through the hole of a spindle head while her abdomen was being massaged. Another method used to ensure the expulsion of the placenta was to tie the umbilical cord to a thread fixed around the woman's hip.
- To avoid hemorrhaging, the uterus was massaged, and the abdomen was tightly bandaged. In cases where this method was unsuccessful, the mother was seated on a hot felt mat that was impregnated with melted fat. Kolbasenko (1899) wrote: "Probably the high temperature of the greased fat caused reflex uterine contractions and therefore stopped the hemorrhaging."
- After delivery was completed, the mother was washed and placed in bed with her abdomen bandaged. She was then left to rest with minimal disturbance.

As a result of the formation of the Soviet system of public health and the development of a maternal and child care preventive health system, as well as the increase in number and training of manpower, the techniques described are no longer in practice in Kazakhstan and are only of educational value.

THE ROLE OF THE MIDWIFE
IN PROVIDING PERINATAL CARE
IN KAZAKHSTAN TODAY

A midwife in Kazakhstan today is a medical officer with special secondary education, who provides preventive/curative and obstetrical/gynecological care.

In the U.S.S.R. midwives are trained at the medical schools, with a three-and-a-half-year training course (as part of an eight-year schooling requirement), and a two-and-a-half-year course (as part of a ten-year schooling requirement).

The main forms of continuing education for midwives are (a) two-month full-time courses in advanced training (as well as extramural training for midwives), and (b) participation in conferences and seminars on problems related to obstetrics and gynecology. Obstetricians/gynecologists regularly examine the theoretical knowledge of midwives, especially of cases where unfavorable outcomes result from gynecological disorders or labor difficulties. Midwives are registered. Study tours for advanced training are organized, annual competitions are held between rural health institutions, and schools are built in connection with hospitals.

A midwife carries out preventive, curative, and health education activities both under the direct control of a physician (at maternity hospitals and obstetrics and gynecological departments of hospitals or clinics for women) or without assistance but under the general supervision of a physician (in rural settings, such as feldsher-midwifery[1] units and collective farm maternity homes).

Professional Rights and Duties of Midwives
at the Various Stages of Perinatal Care

There are five established stages of obstetrical and gynecological care given to the rural population in Kazakhstan.

The first stage of obstetrical and gynecological care is given by midwives (prephysician care) carried out at the feldsher-midwifery units and collective farm maternity homes. The feldsher-midwifery units are normally established in communities with a population of 300–800 (if there is no medical ambulatory unit or hospital within a range of 4–5 km). The personnel of a feldsher-midwifery unit comprises a feldsher, a midwife, and a nurse. Feldsher-midwifery units may be for outpatients alone but may also have beds for women about to begin labor. In Kazakhstan, there are 5453 feldsher-midwifery units, 32 of which have beds for women close to childbirth. Collective farm maternity units were widespread in 1930–40, when the network of maternity hospitals was insufficient. At the maternity home (comprising two or three beds), midwives manage cases of normal labor only. Today, these homes are no longer necessary, as the district hospital

---

[1]*Feldsher*: primary health care worker trained to work where there are no doctors.

provides obstetrical medical care. There are seven collective farm maternity homes at present in Kazakhstan, with a total of twenty-three obstetrical beds.

While the network of collective farm maternity homes and feldsher-midwifery units is on the decline, the number of medical ambulatory units increases. Medical ambulatory units can have only one obstetrician/gynecologist if the workload is minimal. In recent years, the reconstruction and integration of small rural hospitals with district hospitals has become the practice in Kazakhstan.

Providing Obstetrical and Gynecological Care for Women in Rural Areas

A midwife assigned to a feldsher-midwifery unit is a specialist (having graduated from secondary school and possessing the qualifications for midwives-feldshers). The decision to employ or dismiss a midwife is made by the Village Soviet of People's Deputies, in conjunction with the corresponding public health body. An important part of the activities of feldsher-midwifery units is centered on obstetrical care, as well as preventive and curative care for infants, detection of pregnancies at the earliest possible moment, provision of medical care during labor, and supervision of women in their homes who may be close to labor or upon discharge from the hospital.

Midwives instruct women on hygiene during pregnancy, care for infants, proper nursing methods, and prevention of infectious diseases. The outpatient service provided by the feldsher-midwifery unit is mainly of a preventive nature, aimed at avoiding complications during pregnancy. In providing early medical care to pregnant women, the midwife carries out health education work among the women, explaining to them the importance of early visits to the physician or midwife at the start of a pregnancy. Home visits by the midwife provide her with necessary data concerning the women and infants. The midwife can also ensure protection for pregnant women and nursing mothers against work that might prove harmful to their own or their infant's health.

The midwife takes measures to ensure that all pregnant women under her supervision are admitted to the inpatient hospital at the time of delivery. This entails a decision by the midwife as to which inpatient hospital she must refer the pregnant woman to, as well as completing an "individual antenatal record," which she then forwards to an obstetrician-gynecologist in the district hospital.

In addition to curative and preventive care for women and infants, the midwife provides urgent medical care in cases of acute disease and accidents, such as injuries, hemorrhages, and poisoning, and alerts a doctor. In this connection, she also carries out the doctor's instructions, performs early laboratory investigations, and conducts physiotherapeutic treatment.

A midwife in a feldsher-midwifery unit is the primary health care contact for the rural population.

During the final stages of obstetrical-gynecological care, midwives provide curative and preventive care, working under the supervision of obstetrician-gynecologists.

The midwife has the right to apply conservative methods of treatment (under a doctor's order); administer intravenous injections; assist in surgical procedures; perform blood transfusions (under a doctor's supervision); carry out certain obstetrical interventions in situations when the life of the woman in labor is at risk (e.g., removal by hand of the afterbirth, manual examination of the postnatal uterus, and uterine cervix examination in cases of hemorrhage); and to suture first and secondary degrees of perineal rupture.

ORGANIZATION OF SUPERVISION
AND MEDICAL CARE FOR PREGNANT WOMEN

All pregnant women in the region have the possibility of obtaining clinical examinations from an early stage of pregnancy. Registration of these women is done either during the first visit to the women's consultation center or during subsequent examinations.

If the pregnancy is advancing normally, healthy women are recommended to visit the women's consultation center seven to ten days after their first visit to the doctor and to bring the doctor's notes with them. Subsequent visits to the doctor are monthly during the first half of pregnancy, twice a month after the twentieth-week stage of pregnancy, and three to four times a month after the thirty-second-week stage of the pregnancy. In summary, a healthy expectant mother would visit the women's consultation center approximately fourteen or fifteen times during pregnancy. In case of illness or pathological complications in pregnancy not requiring hospitalization, the frequency of examinations is determined by the doctor for each case.

Each pregnant woman should be examined by a therapeutist, stomatologist, otorhinolaryngologist, and other specialists when required.

All examination data, as well as recommendations and prescriptions, are recorded on the individual antenatal record at every visit. After clinical and laboratory surveys (up to twelve weeks of pregnancy), it is decided whether or not the expectant mother falls into a risk group.

During a pregnant woman's visit to the women's consultation center, special inquiries are made concerning the woman's work, her diet, and rest, as well as appropriateness of physical exercise. The obstetrician-gynecologist from the consultation center may provide the woman with a certificate for transfer to easier and less harmful work during her pregnancy.

Antenatal leave is registered during the thirty-second week of the pregnancy, and the doctor informs the woman of the need for more frequent visits to the consultation center during this leave period.

Physio-psychoprophylactic training of pregnant women is carried out by one of the doctors, by one of the midwives from the women's center, or by a highly skilled midwife.

To inform personnel of the obstetrics inpatient hospital about the advancement of a pregnancy and any existing problems, the doctor at the women's clinic gives the patient her case notes at week thirty-two.

The complexity of survey methods used in other various clinics and laboratories depends on whether the woman belongs to a specific risk group. To qualify risk factors in pregnancy, a scoring scheme is used. The high risk group comprises pregnant women with harmful prenatal factors adding up to a score of 10 or more, the medium risk group a score of 5–9, and the low risk group of a score of up to 4. When a score of 10 or more is given, a decision is made to expedite the pregnancy (Table C-1).

Table C-1 Scoring of Perinatal Risk Factors in Kazakhstan

Risk factor	Score
A. Sociobiological	
1. Mother's age < 20 years	2
30–34 years	2
> 40 years	4
2. Father's age > 40 years	2
3. Occupational hazards mother's	3
father's	3
4. Bad habits mother — smoking one packet a day	1
father — excessive drinking	2
5. Emotional stress	1
6. Mother's height and weight 150 cm or less	2
weight no more than 25 kg over norm	2
Total	
B. Obstetric and gynecological history	
1. Parity 4–7	1
8 and more	2
2. Abortions 1	2
2	3
3 and more	4
3. Abortions before the second month or after the last labor	
3 and more	2
4. Premature labor 1	2
2 and more	3
5. Stillbirths 1	1
2 and more	8
6. Neonatal death 1	1
2 and more	7
7. Child development anomalies	3
8. Neurological disorders	2
9. Birth weight (term) < 2500 g or > 4000 g	2
10. Infertility 2–4 years	2
5 years and more	4
11. Uterine cicatrix	3
12. Uterine/ovarian tumors	3
13. Isthico-cervical insufficiency	2
14. Uterine developmental defects	3
Total	
C. Extragenital disorders	
1. Cardiovascular heart disease without circulation disorder	3
heart disease with circulation disorder	10
hypertensive disease, 1–3 degrees	2-8-10
vegeto–vascular dystonia	2

Table C-1   Scoring of Perinatal Risk Factors in Kazakhstan (*Continued*)

Risk factor	Score
C. Extragenital disorders (*continued*)	
2. Kidney disorders before pregnancy	3
during pregnancy	4
adrenal gland disorder	7
3. Endocrinopathies diabetes	10
diabetes (relatives)	1
thyroid gland disorder	7
4. Anemia—Hb 9-10-11	4-2-1
5. Coagulopathies	2
6. Myopia/other eye disorders	2
7. Chronic specific infections	3
8. Acute infections in pregnancy	2
Total	
D. Pregnancy complications	
1. Apparent early toxicosis	2
2. Late toxicosis hydrops gravidarum	2
nephropathy, 1–3 degrees	3-5-10
pre-eclampsia	11
eclampsia	12
3. Hemorrhage in the first and second halves of pregnancy	3-5
4. PH and ABO isosensibilization	5-10
5. Hydramnios	4
6. Oligoamnios	3
7. Pelvic presentation	3
8. Multiple pregnancy	3
9. Prolonged pregnancy	3
10. Malpresentation	3
Total	
E. Fetal state estimation	
1. Fetal hypotrophy	10
2. Fetal hypoxia	4
3. Estriol content of urine 4.9 mg/d at 30 weeks	34
12.0 mg/d at 40 weeks	15
4. Water changes revealed by amnioscopy	8
Total	

CONCLUSION

Bearing in mind the importance of the health of future generations, all these measures are aimed at improving the state of health of both mother and fetus from as early in pregnancy as possible. The network of obstetric institutions, which is broadly developed in the republic, makes it possible for all pregnant women to be under the care of medical officers. The primary clinical examination of pregnant women determines the type of service they require. Apart from the provision of care by both doctors and specialists to the rural population in recent years, the role of midwives (especially at feldsher-midwifery units, where the midwife provides preventive care not only for women and babies but also for the entire population of the sector) has been of utmost importance.

Recommendations

1 The character and level of midwifery training should be allowed to encompass the sphere of the midwife's duties in assisting healthy pregnant women and women in labor. This applies especially to midwives working in rural areas, where they are the main providers of primary health care for the population.

2 In providing curative and preventive care, midwives should be guided by uniform regulations dealing with basic issues of obstetrics and gynecology.

3 The workload of midwives should be planned in accordance with the stages of medical care provision.

Index

197